NOT JUST A PERIOD

Reclaim Your Cycle, Harness Your Hormones
and Take Control of Your Health

DR HAZEL WALLACE

NOT JUST A PERIOD

Reclaim Your Cycle, Harness Your Hormones
and Take Control of Your Health

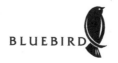

BLUEBIRD

First published 2025 by Bluebird
an imprint of Pan Macmillan
The Smithson, 6 Briset Street, London EC1M 5NR
EU representative: Macmillan Publishers Ireland Ltd, 1st Floor,
The Liffey Trust Centre, 117–126 Sheriff Street Upper,
Dublin 1, D01 YC43
Associated companies throughout the world
www.panmacmillan.com

HB ISBN 978-1-0350-4959-2
TPB ISBN 978-1-0350-4961-5

Poem credit [To Come]

Pan Macmillan does not have any control over, or any responsibility for,
any author or third-party websites referred to in or on this book.

1 3 5 7 9 8 6 4 2

A CIP catalogue record for this book is available from the British Library.

Typeset in Kepler by Jouve (UK), Milton Keynes
Printed and bound by CPI Group (UK) Ltd, Croydon, CR0 4YY

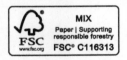

Visit **www.panmacmillan.com/bluebird** to read more about all our books
and to buy them. You will also find features, author interviews and
news of any author events, and you can sign up for e-newsletters
so that you're always first to hear about our new releases.

Poem in praise of menstruation
by Lucille Clifton

if there is a river
more beautiful than this
bright as the blood
red edge of the moon   if

there is a river
more faithful than this
returning each month
to the same delta   if there

is a river
braver than this
coming and coming in a surge
of passion, of pain   if there is

a river
more ancient than this
daughter of eve
mother of cain and of abel   if there is in

the universe such a river   if
there is some where water
more powerful than this wild
water
pray that it flows also
through animals
beautiful and faithful and ancient
and female and brave

Dedication

For anyone who has ever felt confused about, or
been made to feel ashamed of, their menstrual cycle – this
book is a step towards reclaiming that narrative
and embracing your power.

Contents

Part 1
Get To Know Your Cycle

Part 2
Living Alongside Your Cycle

Part 3
Getting Support

About me

Hello, I'm Dr Hazel – former NHS medical doctor and women's health nutritionist.

Many people may know me from social media as The Food Medic, where, since 2012, I have made it my mission to provide evidence-based nutrition and health information through my books, website and social media.

However, in more recent years, I have dedicated my focus to women's health because, as a woman and a health provider to many other women, I have realized that our health needs are underserved and overlooked.

I wrote my last book, *The Female Factor: making women's health count – and what it means for you*, to raise awareness of this. I also wanted to change the accepted narrative that, in medical circles, women are simply 'small men', and argue that they should instead be seen and understood in their own unique way. I hoped this book would be the solution, and while it helped many, it actually sparked an even bigger conversation and opened my eyes to the scale of the problem when it comes to menstrual health.

Since its publication in 2022, many women continue to flood to my DMs and inbox to share their collective experience of struggling with distressing menstrual cycle symptoms and feeling dismissed by healthcare professionals who have led them to believe it's just a normal experience of having a period.

You may be surprised to hear about the number of women who

use their annual leave up as menstrual leave, because their cramps are so debilitating, or the number of women who no longer have a period and have been given no explanation as to why, but have been offered the pill instead. Or, more sinisterly, the many women who have struggled for *years* to get a diagnosis for the severe cyclical mood disorder PMDD (premenstrual dysphoric disorder) and were batted away with 'it's just period-related mood swings'.

When getting support from qualified health professionals seems impossible, many women feel like they have no choice but to take their menstrual health into their own hands. As a result, they often turn to unqualified menstrual health 'coaches' and self-proclaimed hormonal experts on platforms like TikTok, who make a living teaching us how to balance our hormones with their various green powders and crystals. However, because of the lack of research and trusted voices in this space, the sad reality is that menstrual health and cycle syncing is quickly becoming the latest trend in the wellness industry, and many brands are jumping on the bandwagon, hoping to profit from women who have no one else to turn to.

The irony is not lost on me that, as a content creator, I spend a lot of my time undoing the harm caused by social media. Often, when women first come to me in my nutrition clinic, they will be on a whole host of 'women's health' supplements that they've been encouraged to buy through targeted advertisements, or following restrictive diets because they came across a video claiming carbs cause PCOS (polycystic ovary syndrome), or that dairy worsens endometriosis.

The good news is that with the right nutrition support, alongside usual medical care, we can improve symptoms, long-term health and quality of life of the women living with these conditions. I've achieved this first-hand with my clients (and with my own menstrual cycle), but I want that transformation to be possible for all women.

Alongside my team, we have been conducting research through

surveys and focus groups to understand the scale of the problem and give women a platform to share their experiences of their menstrual cycles and the support (or lack thereof) they've received. You will find their stories and the stats from this research peppered throughout the book – and if you helped to contribute, I am hugely grateful.

Over the last few years, we've witnessed a huge drive to raise awareness and educate the masses on the menopause, with documentaries like Davina McCall's *Sex, Myths and the Menopause* and the appointment of the first Menopause Employment Champion by the British government. It has been incredible to see the menopause creep to the top of our health, and this is exactly what I believe needs to happen wit menstrual health. It's not just about the treatment of menstrual disorders, but also education on how we can optimize our health throughout the cycle.

There are lots of books out there that tell us what happens after our periods stop, but little to help us live happily alongside our cycle, rather than simply surviving each month and dreading the next.

This is why I wrote this book. My goal is to help fill the knowledge gap regarding the menstrual cycle and raise awareness in society and among healthcare professionals that the menstrual cycle is not just a period, and can actually impact all aspects of a person's life.

With the right education, awareness and support, we can help women reclaim their cycle, harness their hormones and take control of their health.

Introduction

1.9 billion people on this planet menstruate and, on average, each has a period every 28 days (give or take), from around age 13 to 51, totalling 456 periods over a lifetime.[1]

Just let that sink in.

What we call a 'period' is just the bleeding phase, but *so* much more happens across the remaining 23 (or so) days of your cycle.

Despite the fact that we spend the majority of our lives in any one phase of our menstrual cycle, results from England's 'Women's Health – Let's talk about it' survey found that fewer than a fifth of women feel they have enough information on menstrual wellbeing.[2]

I'm (almost) sure you know this already, but just in case . . . sharks won't attack you if you go swimming on your period, eating lemons won't delay your period and, yep, you can still get pregnant if you have sex during your period.

While some of these (actual) myths might seem amusing, they contribute to the stigma and shame around periods, which can be incredibly damaging for many girls, women and people who menstruate globally. Stigma often reinforces cultural beliefs that portray menstruation as something shameful, rather than acknowledging it as a natural bodily function. Even today in developed countries, periods are frequently considered inappropriate or embarrassing to talk about, with euphemisms like 'Shark Week' (UK), 'Erdbeerwoche' or 'Strawberry Week' (Germany), 'La semaine Ketchup' (France) and 'Aunt Flo' (US) used to soften the subject. In other communities, the stigma can take a darker turn, where women on their period are considered 'unclean' and forbidden from touching food or crops, or even socially excluded or exiled from their homes.[3]

For many in low- and middle-income countries (LMICs), this stigma isn't just about embarrassment – it's rooted in fear, leading to severe social and physical consequences. For example, in Nepal, women and girls forced to stay in unsafe 'Chhaupadi' huts during menstruation have faced poor sanitation, lack of access to clean water, sexual abuse, and even attacks from wild animals. This not only impacts their physical safety, but also affects their mental health, leading to increased risks of anxiety, depression, infections, and missing school.[4]

Menstruation is more than just a personal issue; it's a critical health and education concern that impacts us all, and we need to address it with empathy, whether we menstruate or not. In homes, schools, workplaces and beyond, it's time to break the silence. Everyone deserves the right to be informed about their bodies – and no one should have to live in shame over or feel in the dark about what's happening to their body every month.

Think back to when you got your very first period, or maybe in Sex ED class. You might have learned about how periods arrive roughly every month, and maybe you were told how to use a sanitary towel, or how you shouldn't leave the same tampon in for too long, but were you told how and why our bodies change throughout the cycle? Why our cravings and hunger become insatiable the days before our period, or why our skin suddenly breaks out just when we thought we had it under control? No, me neither.

We were never taught that, apart from reproduction, our menstrual cycles, and the hormones that control them, impact many aspects of our health including our nutritional needs (and cravings!), how strong and energized we feel, and how well we sleep – even down to how our gut works!

This is why *it's not just a period* – it's so much more.

Not only have we kept girls and women in the dark about their bodies, but we've come to accept that any menstrual-related symptoms, like cramps, breakouts and bloating, are simply something we must endure, because it's 'just a period'.

This normalization of women's pain and acceptance of these symptoms is holding us back in life and hindering our ability to progress through education and the workplace. As part of my research for this book, I conducted a survey to explore how the menstrual cycle truly impacts women's daily lives, including their work and relationships. Of the 4,735 people who completed the survey, 91 per cent said that their work is disrupted by their menstrual cycle and, on days when people attend work or university/college while experiencing symptoms, 76 per cent report their concentration being impacted.[5] Research suggests that this presenteeism – that is, working through period-related symptoms like pain or heavy bleeding – causes 9 days of lost productivity for women annually.[6] Even when women do take time off because of symptoms (and our report found that 32 per cent had in the last 12 months), often it's at our expense, because we are either using up our annual leave days or taking it as unpaid leave.

At this point, you might be thinking (rightly, in my opinion): 'But it's the 21st century, *why* is it this way?'

I've been thinking the same and, from years of speaking to women about this, I firmly believe that many women, and girls, feel the need to 'endure' debilitating symptoms month-on-month because as a society we have been normalizing the pain and discomfort of menstruation for so long. But here's the thing: just because something is *common* does not make it *normal* – nor does it mean it's something we shouldn't be concerned about. I've heard from women who have waited eight or more years for a diagnosis of endometriosis, despite being in debilitating pain, because they were led to believe their pain was normal – be that by their teachers in school, friends they spoke to, or health professionals.

In truth, we've all been brainwashed into thinking that menstrual pain is somehow much easier to tolerate, much more acceptable, than any other pain.

Unfortunately, when women do ask for help from health professionals, more often than not they're left feeling dismissed and unsupported – and many end up in my Instagram DMs. While I don't claim to have all the answers, the reason they come to me is because they have no one else to turn to. In fact, in our research survey we found that 38 per cent of people turn to social media influencers for advice regarding their menstrual cycle – but only 13 per cent say it's their preferred source of support. I don't say this to throw my peers under the bus, and I don't believe doctors are intentionally dismissing or 'gaslighting' women, but rather it's a reflection of our limited understanding and attitudes towards menstruation and pain.

On a personal level, it took me two years to get a diagnosis of PCOS because I was told that I didn't 'fit the PCOS picture', despite the fact I was suffering with acne, excessive facial hair growth and my periods were incredibly irregular. Even as a medical doctor, I had to advocate for myself and fight for blood tests and an ultrasound which finally confirmed the diagnosis of PCOS. While the diagnosis was incredibly upsetting, part of me felt relief and validated after months of being told that what I was experiencing was 'normal'.

Unfortunately, this response from healthcare professionals not only delays further access to healthcare and treatment, but it can also lead women to doubt their own experiences and perception of pain. Many come to believe that *'it's all in my head'* and that *'I must have a low pain threshold'*.[7] This is not just true of menstrual-related pain but, in general, even though women more frequently report pain to a healthcare provider, they're also more likely to have their pain dismissed as 'emotional' or 'psychogenic' (i.e., 'not real') compared to a man.[8][9][10] Not only is their pain less likely to be taken seriously, but they're also less likely to be given painkillers for their pain, and when they are, they have to wait longer for them.[11]

Gender biases are one barrier to women receiving adequate care, but our lack of research and education into women's health conditions is another. A measly 2.5 per cent of publicly funded research is dedicated to female reproductive health, despite the fact a third – *a third!* – of women will experience a reproductive or gynaecological health issue in their lives.[12] Compare this to erectile dysfunction, which affects 19 per cent of men and has *five times* more research than premenstrual syndrome, which affects up to 90 per cent of women.[13]

The previous British government pledged to do better when it launched the first-ever Women's Health strategy in 2022, with plans and promises to support more research addressing women's health conditions. The strategy also called for mandatory training in women's health for new doctors in 2024/2025.[14] I've often been asked, 'Is it enough?', and while I applaud the *ambitions* for the strategy, I believe that right now, we need less ambition, more action.[15] At the time of writing, it remains to be seen whether the new government will put any further policies in place.

The bottom line is: the lack of awareness and understanding of menstrual health issues stems from the lack of research in this space. We have decades and decades of research that discounts the female body and simply assumes that we are 'little men'. This means we're basically leaving women's health largely up to guesswork – especially when it comes to the menstrual cycle.

That said, slowly but surely, more and more researchers are waking up to the significant influence that the menstrual cycle has on our health beyond reproduction, from immunity and cardiovascular health to gut function and even the speed of our metabolism.

In fact, many are calling on the menstrual cycle to be labelled the fifth vital sign because it gives us so much insight into our overall health, if we know to listen.[16] Unfortunately, many of us don't even consider our menstrual cycle until there's an issue with it. That said, even if you're one of the lucky ones who has sailed through your periods drama-free since puberty, there is still so much to learn – and so much to gain – from an understanding of this aspect of women's health.

And I'm going to show you why.

As you work through this book, you will learn the power of your hormones and how they're here to help, not hinder you. You'll realize that sometimes minor tweaks to your lifestyle during certain phases of our cycle can make a big difference, like upping your oily fish intake during menstruation, practicing yoga to ease PMS, and optimizing your sleep habits after ovulation.

I truly believe that women's potential is limited by the fact that we've not been told enough about our bodies, so I've made it my mission to change that. With the right knowledge, tools and support, you can regain control of and, better yet, live in tune with your cycle to maximize your energy, reduce your symptoms, boost your productivity and make the most of your life.

My aim with this book is simple: to help you feel empowered, not held back, by your menstrual cycle.

By the end, you will have an gained an understanding of:

* Your unique female physiology, so you can begin to reconnect with your menstrual cycle and deepen your relationship with your body
* What's normal and what's not, so you can spot red flags and challenge your expectations of what you should (and shouldn't) 'put up with' (FYI, periods should never be *that* painful)
* How to optimize your health and performance across the cycle by adjusting your nutrition, movement and sleep, right down to your skincare
* How to navigate changes and fluctuations in body image, libido and mood across the menstrual cycle

✳ How to speak to partners, family and health professionals to advocate best for yourself and your needs

In short, this is the book you'll wish you had been given when you got your first period.

A NOTE ON SEX/GENDER TERMINOLOGY USED IN THE BOOK

Sex and gender are often used interchangeably, but they are different.

✳ **Sex** refers to the biological and physiological differences between males and females; that is, genetics (X X and X Y chromosomes), reproductive organs and hormones. Sex is typically assigned at birth, but it can be changed through medical procedures and hormone treatments. Intersex people are born with sex characteristics (such as sexual anatomy, reproductive organs, hormonal patterns and/or chromosomal patterns) that do not fit typical binary notions of male or female bodies

✳ **Gender** is a social, psychological and cultural construct and relates to the behaviours and attributes expected by different societies and cultures based on their understanding of what it is to be 'masculine' or 'feminine'. People may identify as male, female, agender, or non-binary. Gender can align with one's sex assigned at birth (cisgender) or differ from it (transgender).

In this book, I strive to use these terms correctly. However, even in the research, sex and gender are often (incorrectly) used interchangeably and, as both our sex and gender influence our health and access to healthcare, it can be difficult to quantify the exact contributions of each.

This book focuses on women and those assigned female at birth. When I use the terms 'women' or 'females,' I am referring to women with female reproductive anatomy who identify as women, unless stated otherwise. However, not all cisgender women have a menstrual cycle, and not all people who have a menstrual cycle are cisgender women.

As a cisgender, white female, I also recognize that my experiences may not represent all women's experiences.

Part 1

Get To Know Your Cycle

When people use the term 'cycle', they often mean their period, but it's *so much* more than just a bleed. This is why I called this book *Not Just a Period*, because between puberty and the menopause you will, at any point, be experiencing one phase of this monthly cycle. While the period is one phase, across the remaining days of the cycle your hormones continue to ebb and flow, which can have direct and indirect effects on your strength, energy, nutrition, mood and sleep.

So, let's introduce the menstrual cycle again, because if your first introduction to periods was anything like mine, we've got a lot to go over . . .

'I basically learned about my period, kind of in my late 20s, early 30s, on social media. And now I feel like it's actually quite a bonding experience, because all of my friends are doing the same thing, because none of us were taught it at school. And now we finally understand our bodies. It's like one of our favourite things to talk about, and we are able to support each other better . . . And in that sense, I think it genuinely has made my friendships deeper, because I would say most of my friends struggle in some capacity throughout their cycle, in different ways.' – **Ava, 31**

Overview of the menstrual cycle

We experience our first period, or menstrual cycle, at puberty and go through this cycle 456 times (on average) until we reach menopause – for many, that's almost 40 years of life. So it goes without saying that it's in our best interest to be informed about what's going on in our bodies across the cycle so that we can be better prepared and feel less blindsided by our hormones from month to month.

The menstrual cycle starts with the first day of bleeding (the period) and ends the day before the next menstrual period. You will read in textbooks that each menstrual cycle is 28 days long, but real-world averages suggest that only 16 per cent of women have a 28-day cycle.[1] Anything between 21 to 35 days is considered 'normal', but it's also normal for your cycle length to change over time (decreasing as we get older) and also vary along with factors such as ethnicity, high body mass index (BMI) and lifestyle factors, such as stress and smoking.[2]

We can divide the menstrual cycle into two main phases: the follicular and luteal phases, with ovulation sandwiched in between (see diagram below). All of this is orchestrated by hormones produced by the brain and the ovaries (see box on page XXX).

The follicular phase

The follicular phase starts from day one of the cycle (the first day of bleeding) and ends with ovulation, so it's easy to assume that this phase is 14 days long. However, real-world averages suggest it's more like 17–18 days in length.[3] Often, people refer to the follicular phase as a separate phase *after* the period, when in fact, the period (known as menstruation) occurs during the early follicular phase.

During a period (when bleeding occurs), the hormones oestrogen and progesterone are at their lowest and the lining of the womb (endometrium) begins to shed. To help facilitate this, the endometrium releases compounds called prostaglandins that cause smooth muscle contractions, expelling the menstrual blood and old endometrial cells. Unfortunately, this is why most of us experience pain and cramping in the days leading up to and during a period.

While this explanation may gross some people out, the process is actually pretty incredible when we consider that most wounds

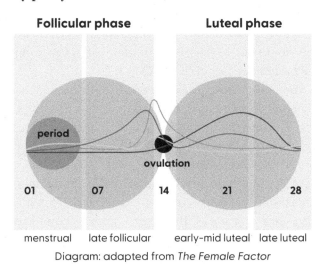

Diagram: adapted from *The Female Factor*

take 4–6 weeks to repair, and often leave a scar, whereas during menstruation, the lining of the womb is shed and goes through a similar repair and regeneration process to any healing process in the body, except that it happens within 5 days, leaves no scars, and happens over and over again for decades.[4] The female body is simply amazing.

Menstruation, or the period, lasts on average 5 days, but can vary between 3–8 days in length. It's common to 'spot' in the days leading up to the period, which is essentially a very small amount of bloody discharge that shouldn't require the use of period products (although this definition can be confusing, as many people still choose to use panty liners when spotting!). You might also notice that the colour of the blood changes as the period progresses, becoming typically darker or brown in colour at the start and end of your period. This is simply because the flow of blood is slower at these times, so it takes longer to exit your body, which gives it more time to oxidize and turn brown.

During the follicular phase, a part of the brain called the hypothalamus releases a hormone called gonadotropin-releasing hormone (or GnRH for short), which stimulates the pituitary gland (another area in the brain) to release follicle-stimulating hormone (FSH). (You don't have to remember all of these hormones, but if you would like to refer back to their roles, I've popped them in a handy reference box on page XXX.)

FSH stimulates the ovaries to develop follicles, which are fluid-filled sacs each containing an egg. The developing follicles produce oestrogen, causing the lining of the womb to build back up. One of these follicles becomes the dominant follicle and is the 'chosen one' to be released at ovulation.

The rising oestrogen levels signal to the brain to release a second hormone, called luteinizing hormone (LH), which surges and causes you to ovulate. The egg then surfs (quite literally) on little finger-like projections called fimbriae from an ovary to the uterus, where it may or may not be fertilized by a sperm.

The luteal phase

The luteal phase begins at ovulation, and lasts until the start of the next menstrual period. In a textbook cycle, this is 14 days long, but in reality it's often slightly longer or shorter. In fact, a study published in the *British Medical Journal* of just 221 women found their luteal phases to last as little as 7 and as many as 19 days.[5] This is important for those wishing to know when they are ovulating (for conceiving or the avoidance of pregnancy), as we assume ovulation occurs on day 14, but it can happen much earlier or later than that.

Some women experience ovulation pain (known as Mittelschmerz) ranging from a mild ache to pretty intense pain. As it's one-sided, and often found on the right of the body, it can sometimes be misdiagnosed as acute appendicitis.[6] If you're someone who finds this pain severe, and over-the-counter painkillers are not helping, you can speak to your doctor about hormonal contraception that prevents ovulation, such as the pill or implant.

Not everyone experiences ovulation pain, but you can figure out if you've ovulated by a few other methods:

* **Cervical mucus:** Around ovulation, you may notice that your discharge increases in volume and might appear like 'egg white' – wet, slippery, clear and stretchy.
* **Basal body temperature:** There's a small rise in body temperature after ovulation takes place. Multiple factors influence body temperature, however, so for the greatest accuracy, make sure to take your temperature at the same time every day, when you wake up, before you eat or drink anything.
* **Ovulation symptoms:** Some women experience physical symptoms around ovulation, such as breast tenderness or pain, but they are not wholly reliable methods of predicting ovulation.

* **Tracking**: I'm a huge advocate of menstrual cycle tracking, using an App or physical diary, and it can absolutely help in working out where you are at in your cycle, but not everyone ovulates on day 14 and, as we've seen, ovulation can vary by 10 days between women.[7] Menstrual trackers are an insightful tool, but remember they rely on algorithms, not magic. Treat them as a guide to understanding your body's patterns – not a rulebook to live by.

* **Ovulation prediction kits**: These work by measuring the LH surge before ovulation, and can be helpful if you're trying to conceive. While this method has the greatest accuracy of all those listed here, they're not always reliable in people with PCOS (who often have elevated levels of LH anyway), so 'false positive' results may be obtained. Also, if you have an irregular cycle, it can be really difficult to decide when to use them.

While you only ovulate once per cycle, it is possible to release more than one egg at a time. When this happens, there is the potential to conceive non-identical twins if both eggs are fertilized. It's also possible not to ovulate at all, even if you have a bleed that month. This is known as an **anovulatory** cycle. It is not uncommon for this to happen occasionally, especially in girls who have just started their periods or in women approaching menopause. It is also more common in those with conditions like polycystic ovary syndrome (PCOS) and hypothalamic amenorrhoea. I'll explore both of these conditions in more detail on pages XX and XX.

After ovulation, the follicle that released the egg transforms into a temporary yet vital structure called the corpus luteum, which plays a central role in the menstrual cycle. This 'upgraded' follicle now produces progesterone and smaller amounts of oestrogen.

Progesterone levels peak about halfway through the luteal phase, preparing the womb lining for a pregnancy. Oestrogen levels, which initially drop after ovulation, rise again and then, like progesterone, also peak in the middle of this luteal phase.

If an egg is fertilized, progesterone from the corpus luteum supports the early pregnancy; if not, the corpus luteum eventually gives up and degrades, and progesterone and oestrogen levels drop. This hormone drop causes the lining of the endometrium to fall away and – yep, you got it – it's time for another period.

HORMONES OF THE MENSTRUAL CYCLE

The key hormones of the menstrual cycle are oestrogen, progesterone, follicle-stimulating hormone (FSH), luteinizing hormone (LH), gonadotropin-releasing hormone (GnRH) and testosterone. Beyond reproduction, these hormones also influence our health in other ways and have an effect on how our body functions. You will become very familiar with the 'hero hormones' oestrogen and progesterone, as they appear in every chapter, but feel free to dog-ear this page to come back to whenever you need to.

HERO HORMONES

Oestrogen: Oestrogen, produced by the ovaries, is a key player in the menstrual cycle and overall reproductive health. It not only helps thicken the womb's lining (endometrium), but also regulates the production of other hormones like luteinizing hormone (LH) and follicle-stimulating hormone (FSH). This role is essential for ovulation and the menstrual cycle: without oestrogen, the body wouldn't be able to properly regulate the development of follicles or the timing of ovulation, which are essential for releasing a mature egg for potential fertilization.

Beyond reproduction, oestrogen also keeps bones strong, protects heart health, boosts brain function and mood, influences sleep quality, improves skin and hair health, supports muscle function and repair, regulates the immune system, and affects sexual desire.

Progesterone: Progesterone prepares the womb lining for pregnancy after ovulation, thickening it so that a fertilized egg can implant itself. If pregnancy occurs, progesterone levels continue to rise, helping to maintain the womb lining and support the pregnancy.

If the egg isn't fertilized, progesterone levels drop, which leads to the shedding of the womb lining, i.e., the period.

Beyond reproduction, progesterone (just like oestrogen) helps maintain bone density, impacts sleep quality and enhances skin health. This multi-functional hormone also regulates the immune system, prevents skin ageing, and supports thyroid function, influencing metabolism and energy levels.

THE SIDEKICKS

Gonadotropin-releasing hormone (GnRH): Produced by the area in the brain called the hypothalamus, this hormone signals to another part of the brain called the pituitary gland to release the hormones FSH and LH, which are crucial for regulating the menstrual cycle.

Follicle-stimulating hormone (FSH): FSH helps ovarian follicles grow and mature, each containing an egg. This is essential for ovulation and the production of oestrogen.

Luteinizing hormone (LH) : LH triggers the release of an egg from the ovary (ovulation) and stimulates the production of oestrogen and progesterone.

Testosterone: Testosterone is often not mentioned in relation to the menstrual cycle, but, in women, 25 per cent of testosterone is produced in the ovaries, and it plays a role in the menstrual cycle by helping to develop the follicles. Testosterone levels rise slightly during the follicular phase, contributing to sexual desire, and generally decrease during the luteal phase.

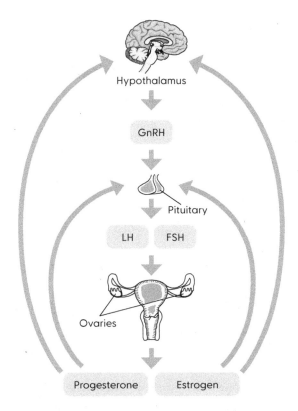

The Hypothalamic-Pituitary- Ovarian-Axis Adapted from "The Menstrual Cycle A Biological Marker of General Health in Adolescents" by V. B. Popat, 2008, *Annals of the New York Academy of Sciences*, 2008 Jul 1;1135:43–51.[8]

Tracking your cycle

When we discuss the menstrual cycle, it's easy to assume that everyone's follows the same textbook pattern; that is, 28 days long, with ovulation happening on day 14. However, as we have discussed, this is essentially the 'Instagram' and not the 'reality' of what happens in real life. Not only do we see variation between people, but we also see variation between cycles, so the best way to figure out what's normal for you is to track your cycle.

Tracking can be done on a very basic level by marking the start and end of your period. Over time, you'll be able to work out how many days your period usually lasts (day 1 of bleeding to the final day of bleeding) and how long your menstrual cycle typically is (day 1 of bleeding to the final day before the next period). With this information, you will be able to roughly know when your next period will come – keeping in mind that the length of periods and amount of days between cycles can vary even between cycles (especially if you've experienced physical or emotional stress or a change in routine).

Another way of tracking your cycle is making use of the number of period-tracking apps that have emerged over the last couple of years. Not only will they track the length of your period and menstrual cycle, they will also identify what day you're likely to ovulate, as well as your 'fertile window'. You can also usually track symptoms and, from there, identify patterns in your cycle.

Benefits of menstrual cycle tracking

* Allows you to be prepared for your next period
* Teaches you what *your* normal is and helps you to identify any red-flag symptoms (such as irregular cycles or bleeding between periods)
* Helps to inform conversations with your doctor and other health care providers
* Can assist with conceiving or avoiding pregnancy.
* Allows you to understand what is happening in your body during each menstrual cycle phase and how to best support it (more on this in part 2!)

In a survey of women's experiences of using period-tracking apps, the majority said the tool made them feel 'prepared' (53 per cent), while some said it helped them feel 'in control' (49 per cent) and 'informed' (37 per cent).[1] However, apps aren't always accurate, and in the same survey, 55 per cent said their period started earlier, and 72 per cent said it started later, than the app predicted. Another review of 140 menstrual tracking apps showed that 22 per cent contained inaccuracies (in content, tools or both).[2] The reason this is important to highlight is that I know many women use these tools for family planning and preventing pregnancy, but, unfortunately, these apps have a high failure rate when used as the only form of contraception[3] – so do use them with caution, if you had that in mind.

TLDR: Menstrual tracking apps are fantastic for body awareness and spotting changes, but not 100 per cent accurate as a method of contraception.

If you're on a form of hormonal contraception and wonder if you can or should track your cycle too, the answer is yes! While you won't experience the same hormonal fluctuations of a 'natural' cycle, you may experience some cyclical variation, depending on the type of contraception. It's also still useful to track symptoms you may experience, such as fluctuations in energy, mood, libido, motivation, performance etc., as these can help you make informed choices around the most suitable hormonal contraception method for you.

CONSIDERATIONS WHEN CHOOSING A PERIOD-TRACKING APP

Privacy and data security: Ensure the app has a clear privacy policy regarding how your data is stored, used and shared. Look for apps that store data locally on your device or use encryption.

Free vs. paid: Determine whether you need a free app or if you're willing to pay for premium features. Some apps offer basic tracking for free but charge for advanced features like fertility predictions or health reports.

Features: Check if the app allows you to track more than just your period, such as symptoms, moods, ovulation and lifestyle factors (e.g., exercise, diet). Some apps have specialized features for teenagers and athletes, etc.

Integration: Check compatibility with other health and fitness apps you use.

Accuracy: No app will be 100 per cent accurate, as the human body can be unpredictable at times. Apps approved by organizations like the FDA, however, or those that include medically reviewed information, may provide more accurate guidance and predictions.

Cycle regularity: If you have a regular menstrual cycle, the app's predictions are likely to be more accurate. However, for those with irregular cycles, predictions will likely be less reliable.

What's normal, what's not

Despite the heading of this section, there is no such thing as a 'normal' menstrual cycle – every cycle is unique and can fluctuate across a lifetime, especially when periods start (puberty) and are coming to an end (perimenopause). Some women also notice their menstrual cycle changes after pregnancy. I explore how periods might change during these different life stages on page XX.

All that said – there are some generally accepted characteristics of a healthy period, as well as some red flags you shouldn't ignore.

Menstrual cycle 'green' flags	Menstrual cycle 'red' flags
➤ Cycle length between 21 and 35 days ➤ Period length between 3 and 7 days ➤ No bleeding between periods or after sex ➤ Very little cramping ➤ Menstrual symptoms and flow are not interfering with day-to-day life	➤ Heavy periods ➤ Painful periods ➤ Bleeding between periods or after sex ➤ Irregular or absent periods ➤ Cyclical, severe mood changes related to menstrual cycle ➤ Any menstrual cycle symptom causing significant disruption to daily life (i.e., work/school, social life, relationships)

Basically, there are a lot of things that can go wrong with your period. It may disappear or become irregular, it may be extremely heavy or very painful, or you may bleed when you shouldn't (i.e., between your periods, after sex, and after the menopause).

Unfortunately, this topic deserves a whole book to itself, so this next section will be a bit of a whistle-stop tour through the red-flag symptoms. However, your biggest takeaway from this section should be: if it's not normal for you, it's worth chatting with your doctor.

Heavy periods (menorrhagia)

Let's start with heavy periods, and how heavy is *too* heavy.

Case Study: Grace

Grace, a 20-year-old student, had always thought it was normal to go through a tampon every hour, often using a pad at the same time. It wasn't until she chatted with a friend at uni, complaining how much money she had spent on tampons that month, that she realized most people don't experience such heavy periods. That conversation made Grace realize her periods were a lot heavier than other women's, and prompted a discussion with her doctor. She was diagnosed with iron deficiency anaemia, which was corrected with supplements, and was offered medication to reduce her flow. Grace's story shows how important it is to talk openly about periods, because one conversation might just help someone recognize something isn't quite right. While such heavy periods may be common for many women, it's not normal.

If we look at the guidelines,[1] heavy periods can be defined as blood loss of 80ml or more (about half a teacup) and/or bleeding that lasts for more than 7 days.[2] It's very difficult to know how much blood you're losing, and perhaps a more practical definition is one from the National Institute for Health and Care Excellence (NICE), which defines a heavy period as 'excessive blood loss that interferes with a woman's physical, social, emotional and/or quality of life.'[3]

Other signs of heavy periods are:

* Changing a tampon/pad every 1–2 hours, or having to empty a menstrual cup after only a few hours
* Using two types of sanitary products at once
* Passing large blood clots (>2.5 cm. or the size of 10p coin)
* Regularly leaking through to your clothes or bedding
* Avoiding daily activities, like exercise, or taking time off work due to your flow

A lot of women (including you, perhaps?) believe that heavy periods are just bad luck. A recent survey from Wear White Again of 1,000 women who experienced heavy periods found that 62 per cent of them didn't realize that heavy menstrual bleeding (known as *menorrhagia*) is a diagnosable medical condition and instead assumed it was just something they had to put up with.[4] Well, you don't, and there are treatments that can help.

Heavy periods are not only a bit of a nuisance to deal with, but they have direct health consequences, such as iron deficiency anaemia and the fatigue that comes with it. There are also indirect health consequences that come as a result of avoiding social occasions and skipping exercise, out of fear of leaking.

Causes of heavy periods

In about half of reported cases, no cause for the heavy bleeding is found, and this is called dysfunctional uterine bleeding (DUB).

In some cases, heavy periods can be due to any underlying cause, such as:

* Fibroids
* Polyps
* Endometriosis
* Adenomyosis
* Pelvic inflammatory disease (an infection of the female reproductive system, including the womb, fallopian tubes and ovaries)
* Hormonal conditions (such as PCOS)
* Endometrial hyperplasia (thickening of the womb lining) or cancer
* Blood clotting disorders
* Certain medications
* The copper coil
* The very beginning of periods (puberty) or their ending (perimenopause)

Suffice to say, if you have heavy periods, it is important that you are checked to rule out any abnormalities.

Managing heavy periods

Treatment, if required, will depend on the underlying cause (see pages XX and XX for more on this).

If, after testing, no underlying medical cause is found, there are a few options available:

* **Do nothing:** This is only an option if the heavy periods are not interfering too much with normal life.
* **Medication:** There is medicine you can take during your period to reduce bleeding, such as tranexamic acid, naproxen or mefenamic acid.

- **Tranexamic acid**: This helps your blood clot better, which reduces how much you bleed during your period. Basically, it helps your body hold onto blood rather than losing too much. You'd usually take it for 3–5 days during your period.
- **Naproxen and mefenamic acid**: These are anti-inflammatory meds, like ibuprofen, and they work by lowering certain chemicals (prostaglandins) that make your uterus contract and cause bleeding. By calming these chemicals down, you bleed less, and often have less cramping too. You take them during your period for a few days.

✳ **Hormonal contraception**: The hormonal coil or the pill help lighten heavy periods by thinning the womb lining. With some methods such as the hormonal coil (e.g. Mirena) periods may stop altogether.

✳ **Surgery**: This is not a first-line treatment, but it can be an option if the above treatments do not help or are unsuitable.

Painful periods (dysmenorrhoea)

It is very common to experience some discomfort and cramping in the days before and during your period, but an estimated 45–95 per cent of women suffer with very painful periods (known as dysmenorrhoea) that interfere with their day-to-day life. Make no mistake, that's huge. By some estimates, that would mean almost all women have very painful periods, and we're just putting up with it![5]

It might surprise you (or not!) to learn that painful periods are the leading cause of school absences and lost working hours in women.[6] Women with dysmenorrhoea have significantly reduced quality of life, poorer mood and sleep quality, and are less active during their periods than women without dysmenorrhoea.[7] Yet, despite the negative impact of painful periods on women's lives, most don't seek medical attention. Research shows that there are a few reasons for this. Firstly, people might consider their symptoms normal – 'something that comes with the territory'. But another key driver in not seeking help is feeling embarrassed, or not confident that healthcare providers will offer help, even if they do ask for it.[8] For most women, however, menstruation is a normal and healthy part of life – we should be no more ashamed of discussing it with a doctor than we would a headache or a painful knee.

Pain is also subjective and, similar to heavy periods, not easily measured. Even so, if your period pain is causing distress, is associated with other symptoms such as nausea, vomiting or dizziness, or is interfering with activities that you'd usually do when you *don't* have your period, you should definitely speak to your doctor. In Part 3, I've included advice about how to speak to health professionals about your period, which you might find useful in this scenario.

There was an article published in the *Independent* in 2016 with the headline: 'Period pain is officially as bad as a heart attack', and I've seen this claim circulate around social media too. Unfortunately, it doesn't seem to be linked to any published research that I can find. I'm also not sure it's a helpful comparison because, while I don't deny heart attacks are painful, not all those who are having heart attacks come to hospital with the classic, 'elephant-sitting-on-your-chest' pain* you usually hear about, and heart attacks can often feel a bit more like indigestion, which is why many delay seeking help initially. As Dr Jen Gunter wrote in response to the article: 'It would be dangerous for women to think that a heart

---

* Side note: if you do experience central crushing chest pain that doesn't go away, please do go to the hospital!!

attack should be at least as bad as their menstrual cramps'[9] –
period pain, for some, may actually be *worse*!

Causes of period pain

Frustratingly, most often, there is no underlying cause for painful
periods. We call this primary dysmenorrhoea ('primary' means no
other health condition is causing it).

Period pain is thought to be a result of prostaglandins (hor-
mone-like compounds) released by the endometrium (womb
lining) as it starts to shed. These compounds make the uterus
contract, reduce blood flow to the uterus and increase sensitivity
of nerve endings – lowering the pain threshold. If that isn't enough,
they can also act on the nearby gut, causing diarrhoea, nausea and
vomiting. While the link hasn't been definitively proven, research
has found that women with primary dysmenorrhoea have higher
levels of prostaglandins compared to those who don't, and pain
intensity also seems to be proportional to the amount of prostaglandin released.[10]

Painful periods can also be due to underlying medical conditions such as endometriosis, adenomyosis, fibroids, or pelvic
inflammatory disease. This is known as secondary dysmenorrhoea.
If your doctor suspects you have an underlying cause for your
painful periods, they may refer you to a specialist gynaecologist
for further investigations and treatment. Treating secondary dysmenorrhoea depends on the underlying cause, and you can find
out more about the various conditions in the appendix.

Managing period pain

In terms of managing painful periods at home, here are some
methods which have evidence (to varying degrees) behind them:

* **Painkillers:** Non-steroidal anti-inflammatory painkillers
  (NSAIDs), such as ibuprofen, act by blocking prostaglandin
  production and have been shown to be very effective

in relieving period pain.[11] Paracetamol is an alternative painkiller you can try if you cannot take NSAIDs (for example, those with a stomach ulcer, and some people with asthma).

* **Heat therapy:** We all have that friend who is glued to her hot-water bottle during her period – and for good reason. Heat has been shown to be as effective as painkillers, such as NSAIDs and aspirin, for menstrual cramp pain. [12] [13] [14] These studies use heat patches which you can pick up from most pharmacies and some supermarkets.

* **Transcutaneous electrical nerve stimulation (TENS) machine:** This is essentially a small machine that produces a small low-voltage electrical current that interferes with pain signals sent to the brain from the nerves. In the UK, you would normally have to buy a TENS machine, however, as they are not available on the NHS to treat period pain.

* **Exercise:** While it may seem like the least appealing thing to do when you're struggling with period pain, there is some evidence to suggest that moderate exercise may help reduce the intensity and duration of menstrual pain. In particular, yoga seems to be especially effective, likely due to the mind–body connection it integrates into the practice.[15] [16] We discuss this more in Chapter XX.

* **Nutrition and supplementation:** There's not a huge amount of evidence supporting specific dietary changes or supplements that can help with painful periods, but there might be some benefit in the use of omega 3, calcium, vitamin D and magnesium (see page xx for more).

Most women with painful periods have mild pain that they can treat themselves at home. However, if your pain becomes more severe and is interfering with your usual activities, you should see your doctor, who can offer prescription medications and hormonal contraceptives that improve period pain.

Irregular and absent periods

It's very common for women to experience a missed period at some point in their reproductive life, and usually it's nothing to worry about.

If you're pregnant, breastfeeding, or post-menopausal, absent periods are totally normal and can be expected. This is also the case if you are taking contraception or have recently stopped. While the former may seem slightly obvious, some forms of contraception will cause your periods to become very light or stop altogether (one example is the hormonal coil). Even after stopping hormonal contraception, it may take a few weeks for your cycle to return. This should occur within 4 weeks, but it's reasonable to give it 3 months. If it doesn't return by then, it would be wise to speak to your doctor to investigate why, because while the pill doesn't cause amenorrhoea, it can mask underlying conditions that do.

However, if none of the above apply, and your period suddenly disappears or comes less frequently, it's probably a sign from your body that something isn't quite right.

We call it 'primary amenorrhoea' if the person has not had a period by the time of expected puberty, and 'secondary amenorrhoea' if the person previously had a period but has now stopped for 3–6 months in a row. Primary amenorrhoea is rare and affects less than 0.1 per cent of women.[17] It happens for a number of reasons, including hormonal conditions, eating disorders, Turner's syndrome (when a female is born with one X chromosome when there should be two), anatomical variations, chronic illness or as a result of certain medications. There may also be no actual cause, but simply a delay in progressing through puberty.

Secondary amenorrhoea is much more common, affecting an estimated 4 per cent of women. However, when we look at active women in particular, rates skyrocket: up to 56 per cent of cyclists, 40 per cent in triathletes and 31 per cent in gymnasts.[18] Anecdotally, I see it all the time with regular gym-goers and women training for marathons and triathlons (for reasons I'll come on to next).

'Oligomenorrhea' is the term for irregular periods, by which we mean occurring less frequently than every 35 days, or less than 9 periods per year.[19] There is considerable overlap between secondary amenorrhoea and oligomenorrhoea, so I will discuss them together.

Causes of irregular/absent periods

✳ Physiological causes
- Pregnancy
- Lactation (breastfeeding)
- Menopause

✳ Premature ovarian insufficiency (POI)
POI is when the ovaries stop working before the age of 40, and may be due to early menopause, a result of surgery or cancer treatment, genetic conditions, autoimmune conditions. In many cases, however, the cause is unknown.

✳ Functional hypothalamic amenorrhoea (FHA)
FHA is when your periods stop due to stress, excessive exercise, or significant weight loss. This happens because your brain slows down the release of hormones needed for ovulation. (See page xx for more on this.)

✳ Other hormonal causes such as
- PCOS
- Thyroid disorders

✳ Pituitary gland problems
✳ Anatomical reasons

Irregular/missed periods can occur after treatment to the cervix or surgery of the uterus
* Certain medications, surgery, or cancer treatment

* Start and end of reproductive life
Irregular periods are also common just after puberty or just before the menopause.

Periods can also become infrequent and erratic during particularly stressful periods of our lives. One recent example of this, that all of us experienced, was the COVID-19 pandemic. Even during the first lockdown, I was hearing from my patients, friends and colleagues about how their cycles had suddenly gone a bit out of whack. These anecdotal reports were confirmed by research, with some studies reporting as many as 75 per cent of women experiencing changes to their cycle during the pandemic.[20] Interestingly, this particular study found that these changes were not significantly different between participants who had been infected with COVID-19 and those who hadn't – suggesting that societal and lifestyle shifts during the pandemic, such as changes to sleep, stress and exercise behaviour, were largely to blame.[21] We chat more about how stress can impact the menstrual cycle in chapter XXX (page XXX).

Abnormal bleeding patterns

The final red flag when it comes to the menstrual cycle is bleeding when you shouldn't be, i.e. between your periods, after sex, or after the menopause. These patterns of unexpected bleeding are symptoms, rather than diagnoses, and warrant further assessment by a doctor. It can be quite scary if it happens, and often the fear women have is that it's a sign of cancer. While gynaecological cancers can present in this way, however, in most cases the cause is benign.

Bleeding between periods (intermenstrual bleeding)

Bleeding between your periods can be due to many reasons, including:

* Ovulation spotting
* Early pregnancy
* Hormonal fluctuations during the perimenopause
* Missed oral contraception or 'breakthrough' bleeding*
* Physical conditions (such as fibroids and polyps) and infections
* Vaginal dryness
* Cancer of the womb, cervix, vagina or vulva

Bleeding after sex (post-coital bleeding)

Some people may experience spotting after their first time having sex, which is normal. However, consistently spotting after penetrative vaginal sex is not considered normal and is something to speak to your doctor about. Post-coital bleeding might occur due to infection, cervical ectropion,† trauma, vaginal dryness, and in some cases cancer of the cervix or vagina. In younger women, the risk of cancer is very low, but it is always sensible to get any unusual bleeding checked out by your doctor. Cervical cancer is

---

* Breakthrough bleeding is a common side effect of hormonal contraception, especially with low-dose pills, IUDs/coils, and implants, often causing spotting or irregular bleeding in the first few months. While not harmful, persistent or bothersome bleeding should be discussed with your doctor to explore solutions.

† Cervical ectropion is when cells from inside the cervical canal move to the outside of the cervix (the neck of the womb). It's a common condition, not harmful, and often occurs due to hormonal fluctuations caused by pregnancy or birth control.

highly preventable, through HPV vaccination and cervical screening, and highly curable if caught early.

Bleeding after the menopause (post-menopausal bleeding)

Although changes in bleeding are to be expected during perimenopause, if you experience bleeding after you've gone through the menopause (so, bleeding 12 months after your last period), it should be investigated. The menopause is outside the scope of this book, but more information can be found in my previous book, *The Female Factor*.

Cyclical, severe mood changes related menstrual cycle

Many women experience physical and emotional changes around their period, with 90 per cent reporting some premenstrual symptoms like bloating, breast tenderness, breakouts, constipation and minor mood changes. While, for most women, symptoms are mild and manageable, some do have more severe and disruptive symptoms in their luteal phase that interfere with their daily lives.

Premenstrual syndrome (PMS)

PMS affects about 20–40 per cent of women and it refers to a range of physical, emotional and behavioural symptoms that occur 1–2 weeks before the period and subside, or improve, when it starts.[22] Symptoms of PMS include changes in appetite, weight gain, abdominal pain, back pain, lower back pain, headache, swelling and tenderness of the breasts, nausea, constipation, anxiety, irritability, anger, fatigue, restlessness, mood swings and crying.[23]

Premenstrual dysphoric disorder (PMDD)

PMDD is a severe form of PMS, marked by intense mood symptoms such as irritability and depression, emerging 1–2 weeks before menstruation and resolving with its onset. This condition affects 2–8 per cent of women and can make it difficult to work, socialize and maintain relationships. In severe cases, it can also lead to suicidal thoughts.[24]

We explore PMS and PMDD in greater detail in Chapter X.

Premenstrual exacerbation (PME)

Additionally, women with pre-existing mental health conditions, such as depression or bipolar disorder, may experience worsening symptoms in the premenstrual phase, referred to as premenstrual exacerbation (PME).

Your cycle, start to finish

It's normal for your menstrual cycle to change through the decades, from the first menstrual period (known as the menarche) to the last menstrual period (the menopause).

The first period (menarche)

Menarche is the term used to describe a girl's first menstrual period. The average age that this happens in the UK and US is 12, but the normal range is between 9 and 15 years of age – although it can occur earlier and later than this.[1] If periods do not start by age 15 (or age 13 without any other signs of puberty), then you should speak to your doctor.

The first period tends to be painless and usually occurs without warning, which can be pretty stressful, as it often happens in school (when unprepared). Initially, cycles tend to vary in length, lasting fewer than 20 days or longer than 45. This can make it tricky to manage menstrual hygiene, so it's best to always carry some emergency period products in your bag (see more on page xx). By the third year after menarche, 60–80 per cent of menstrual cycles are 21–34 days long, which is typical of adults.[2] [3]

During the first two years after the first period, about half of a girl's menstrual cycles are anovulatory, meaning ovulation hasn't happened and no egg is released.[4] When ovulation is delayed or doesn't happen, either naturally or because of conditions like polycystic ovary syndrome (PCOS), this results in lack of progesterone and excessive oestrogen production from ovarian follicles, causing the womb lining to build up, leading to irregular and often heavy bleeding. While this is common, if periods are very heavy (see page xx for signs), then it's important to speak to a doctor for support and also to rule out bleeding disorders.

After having a baby (postpartum)*

After having a baby, when your periods come back varies and depends largely on whether you're breastfeeding or not:

* If you choose not to breastfeed, your period usually returns within 6–8 weeks of pregnancy.[5]
* If you exclusively breastfeed, your periods may not start again until you start to reduce breastfeeding, but can return anywhere between 4–5 months to 2 years after pregnancy.[6]
* If you bottle-feed or combine breastfeeding and bottle-feeding your baby, you'll tend to start having periods sooner than if you exclusively breastfeed. This can be as soon as 6 weeks after pregnancy.[7]

Breastfeeding can delay your period because of the hormones involved in milk production.[8] Even without a period, you can still ovulate and potentially get pregnant – so keep this in mind if this is something you wish to avoid.[9] [10] [11] However, breastfeeding can be used as an effective form of contraception (known as the lactational amenorrhoea method, or LAM) if the below criteria are met:

---

* It's a difficult reality that not all pregnancies result in live births, but experiencing pregnancy-related period loss also alters your periods. Your period may return within 4 to 8 weeks, but your first period might feel different, and your cycle may also be irregular initially as your body heals – if you're concerned, don't hesitate to reach out to your GP for support.

* Your baby is under 6 months of age
* You are exclusively breastfeeding (at least every 4 hours during the day and every 6 hours at night)
* You are not having periods

If used correctly, the lactational amenorrhea method is 99 per cent effective.[12] This means that 2 women in 100 who use LAM will become pregnant in a year.

When your period does come back, it might be a bit irregular and also heavier at first. It's advised not to use tampons or menstrual cups until after you've had your 6-week postnatal check, and instead use maternity or period pads during this time while your body heals.[13]

Anecdotally, many women tell me how their periods changed after pregnancy – some women experience heavier, longer or more painful periods, while others see their periods improve.

Be careful not to confuse your first period after pregnancy with the vaginal discharge that you experience after giving birth, called lochia, which is often quite bloody, especially in the days after delivery. Lochia generally lasts for about 4 to 6 weeks, but this can vary from person to person. If you notice any signs of infection (like a foul smell) or are losing blood in large clots, tell your midwife or doctor.

Perimenopause

The perimenopause is the transitional period leading up to menopause, often beginning in a woman's forties and lasting several years. During this time the amount of oestrogen produced by the ovaries may begin to fluctuate and you may not ovulate as regularly.

Unlike menopause, it's not always obvious when a woman is going through perimenopause, and that's partly because it doesn't get as much attention and so there's a lack of awareness when it comes to this stage of a woman's reproductive life. During perimenopause, hormones don't just drop in a smooth, predictable way. Instead, they go up and down, making things feel pretty chaotic (see diagram below). Because of this, hormonal blood tests aren't very reliable for figuring out if you're in perimenopause.

These hormonal fluctuations lead to a host of symptoms, the most common being a change to the menstrual cycle, but also hot flashes, vaginal dryness and mood changes. Your periods may come more or less often, be longer or shorter than usual, or be lighter or heavier. Some months you might not get a period. If it's been 12 months since your last period, this is now known as the menopause.

Diagram to follow

Changes in ovarian hormones (oestrogen and progesterone) across the reproductive life cycle of women, from Haufe A, Baker F C, Leeners B. The role of ovarian hormones in the pathophysiology of perimenopausal sleep disturbances: A systematic review. *Sleep Med Rev.* 2022 Dec; 66:101710[14]

Period products

When choosing the right period product, there's no one-size-fits-all answer. Several factors to consider are your flow level, day or night wear, work and activities, and even environmental impacts. Below are some key points to help you decide which products might work best for you throughout your cycle:

* **Flow level:** Make sure the product matches your flow – whether it's light, medium or heavy. This is likely to change throughout your period, so you may find that you need different products for different days of your cycle.
* **Comfort:** Go with what feels best for you. Some people prefer internal options like tampons or menstrual cups, while others feel more comfortable with pads or period underwear.
* **Lifestyle:** Think about your daily routine. If you're active, tampons or menstrual cups might be your go-to, but pads or period underwear could be better for less active days and also when sleeping/resting.
* **Environmental impact:** Some options, such as menstrual cups, cloth pads and period underwear, are more eco-friendly, but they're not always as widely available as other, disposable options.
* **Convenience:** Choose something that's easy to use and change, especially if you're always on the move or don't always have access to private restrooms.
* **Cost:** Think about the long-term cost. Reusable products might cost more upfront, but save money over time, while disposables are cheaper but require regular restocking.

Period product	How to use	Capacity	Change frequency	Pros	Cons
Tampons	Insert into the vagina with an applicator or finger	Light to super plus (depends on size)	Every 4–8 hours, or when saturated	Discrete, suitable for sports and swimming Variety of absorbency levels	Avoid using overnight if sleeping longer than 8 hours
Sanitary towel (pad)	Stick the adhesive side to your underwear	Light to heavy flow (varies by pad thickness and size)	Every 4–6 hours, or when saturated Night-time pads don't need to be changed	Great for overnight use and widely available	Can feel bulky and not suitable for swimming

Period Product	How to use	Capacity	Change frequency	Pro	Con
Panty liners	Stick the adhesive side to your underwear	Discharge to light flow	Every 4–6 hours	Ideal for light flow or spotting at the start/end of a period	Very low absorbency
Menstrual cups	Fold and insert into the vagina. Ensure it opens fully to create a seal. To remove, pinch the base to break the seal and gently pull it out.	Can hold the equivalent of around 2 to 4 regular tampons, depending on the size and brand[15][16]	Every 8–12 hours, depending on flow	Reusable, eco-friendly, long wear time (up to 12 hours), cost-effective over time	Learning curve for insertion/removal, can be messy, not ideal for everyone Using a menstrual cup can risk your coil coming out.[17]

Period Product	How to use	Capacity	Change frequency	Pro	Con
Menstrual discs	Squeeze the sides together to make it the size of a tampon, then insert it pointing down and back into your vagina. Push it back until it sits just behind your pubic bone at a vertical angle, ensuring it completely covers your cervix.	Can hold the equivalent of around 4–5 regular tampons,[18] depending on the brand	Every 8–12 hours, depending on flow	Reusable, eco-friendly, long wear time (up to 12 hours), cost-effective over time Was found to hold the most blood in a study comparing period products[19] Allows for mess-free sex while having a period	Learning curve for insertion/removal, can be messy, not widely available

Period Product	How to use	Capacity	Change frequency	Pro	Con
Period pants	Wear like regular underwear. After use, rinse in cold water before washing, then air dry to maintain absorbency	Light to heavy flow (varies by brand and style)	Can be worn for 8-12 hours or until saturated	Reusable, comfortable, good for overnight use	Expensive upfront, requires frequent washing, was found to hold the least blood in a study comparing period products[20]
Reusable pads	Place the pad in your underwear and snap the wings around the sides to secure it. After use, rinse in cold water and wash with your laundry	Light to heavy flow (varies by pad thickness and size)	Every 4-6 hours	Reusable, eco-friendly, available in various sizes and designs	Requires washing, and can be bulky

A note on period poverty

Period poverty occurs when people can't afford or don't have access to the menstrual products, hygiene facilities, and/or information they need to manage their periods properly. A recent ActionAid report found that more than 1 in 5 women and people who menstruate in the UK are now struggling to afford period products.[21]

When someone can't manage their period comfortably, it can lead to missed days at school or work, health issues, and feelings of embarrassment or shame. If you or someone you know are facing challenges accessing period products, or you want to learn more and how to support, check out the various organization, charities and schemes below:

* **UK Government Period Product Scheme:** Offers free period products to students in schools and colleges across the UK.
* **Period Poverty UK:** Provides assistance and resources for those experiencing period poverty.
* **Freedom4Girls:** Works to break down menstruation stigmas, provides education and distributes period products, with a focus on -sustainable and affordable options.
* **Hey Girls:** An award-winning social enterprise that supplies period products to local authorities and educational institutions, aiming to end period poverty in the UK.

Contraception

922 million women of reproductive age (or their partners) are using some form of contraception[1] – and if that's you, you might be thinking, how does all of the above apply to me?

The good news is that you can absolutely still benefit from reading this book, and in this section, and peppered throughout the book, I will discuss how hormonal contraception impacts your body and influences things like your mood, nutrition and strength.

History of contraception

The first documented reference to what could be described as a condom dates back as far as 3000 BC, in a tale that describes King Minos of Crete reportedly using a goat bladder to protect his wife from 'serpents and scorpions' in his semen (please do not try this one at home).[2] By 1000 AD, Egyptian men purportedly wore coloured linen sheaths as condoms – each colour was used to distinguish status in their social hierarchy, naturally.[3] It wasn't until the 1920s that latex was introduced and used in condoms.[4]

Thirty years later, the first oral contraceptive pill was developed by researchers (and devout Catholics) Gregory Pincus and John Rock, at the urging of Margaret Sanger, a passionate supporter of women's rights (but also a supporter of eugenics).[5] Prescription of the pill was initially restricted to married women only in the UK and to those with 'menstrual disorders' in the USA – where it was not even legal to discuss contraception or prescribe the pill for the indication of contraception until 1969![6] The invention of the pill was a game-changer for many women, giving them control over their reproductive health and letting them plan their careers, education and personal lives with much more freedom. While feminists initially hailed the pill as liberating, some later criticized it as a tool of patriarchal control, questioning why contraception was only a female responsibility and pointing out the male dominance in the medical and pharmaceutical industries.

These first-generation, higher-dose pills raised a lot of safety concerns, so throughout the 1960s and 1970s, new lower-dose pills were introduced to reduce side effects and health risks. Today's pills contain much lower hormone doses and use hormones that are much more pharmacologically specific and focused in their drug effect. During this time we also saw expansion in the variety of contraceptive methods, including the introduction of the progesterone-only pill, the development of IUDs, and emergency contraception. But despite advances in medical research, we have yet to finesse the male pill, and, at the time of writing, the only available male methods of contraception are condoms or a vasectomy. However, research into male contraceptive gels and pills is currently underway, and results have been encouraging so far. The main limiting factor is finding an option that has no-to-low side effects and, of course, funding.

TikTok and pill fearmongering

I think it's amazing that, of all the medications that have been invented in human history, the combined oral contraceptive pill (COCP) is the only pill that is known as 'The Pill'. This shorthand title made it easy for people to refer to the COCP without having to use its full technical name and also emphasized the simplicity and convenience of taking a daily tablet. Over time, as the use of oral contraceptives became widespread, the pill became ingrained in popular culture and language as the go-to reference for this form of contraception.

However, thanks to the widely exaggerated and often incorrect claims that have been made on social media, the pill is currently going through a bit of a rough patch in terms of its public image. And while legitimate concerns and questions about the pill (or any medication we use) are completely valid – and, yes, there are side effects to be aware of – TikTok or #PillTok is not the place to seek this information. While writing this book I stumbled across this dark corner of social media where there are hundreds of videos in which creators are claiming that the pill, and hormonal contraception in general, is damaging our bodies, causing infertility and, as tweeted by Elon Musk, no less, making us 'fat and [doubling] the risk of depression'. The anti-pill brigade seem to feel that that their own experience can be extrapolated to what's best for all women. This excessive fear of hormones has been coined 'hormonophobia', and is 'based on irrational causes such as an overestimation of health risks associated with their use, that was already aroused by the recurring media controversies over hormonal contraception'.[7]

I myself have been labelled a 'pill pusher' for attempting to correct quite damaging and concerning claims related to the pill in the comments section of viral TikTok videos. So, before I go any further, let me be clear: firstly, I am not paid by 'big pharma', and secondly, I am pro informed choice and pro informed decision, meaning I want people who are making any decisions about their body – including the choice to use hormonal contraception or not – to have all the relevant, accurate information, including the benefits and risks, as well as alternatives, before making a decision. I think everyone deserves that right. While social media is not the place to go to receive trusted information (unless from reputable sources *subtle plug*), it's often more accessible than waiting in a queue at the doctor's office. Even when women do manage to bypass the GP's receptionist to share their experiences, they often feel their concerns regarding hormonal contraception are delegitimized and 'not taken seriously'.[8] On the other hand, most doctors in primary care, who are having these conversations, are also only allocated 10 minutes for each patient, which is simply not enough time to counsel someone on their options, the risks and benefits of each, and prescribe.

I think if more women felt fully informed about their options, there would be less fear and anxiety surrounding social media and more trust in the health professionals who prescribe hormonal contraception. A recent review of 42 studies, exploring reasons for rejecting hormonal contraception, found that many were fearful of experiencing side effects and the long-term impact on their health, such as an increased risk of cancer.[9] With that in mind, let's now talk about those potential side effects.

Side effects of the pill

Look, we all know that if you unravel the information leaflet that comes with any medication you're prescribed, you be confronted with a list of potential side effects the length of your arm. The pill is no different. Reading that there is a risk of 'blood clots' or 'cancer' associated with a medication can be pretty alarming, I know. However, what's often missing from these lists, or not illustrated sufficiently, is the *level* of risk that comes with each side effect.

For example, there is a small increased risk of breast cancer while taking the pill, which slowly disappears after you've stopped taking it for 10 years. However, the risk of breast cancer is generally low in women in the age group who are taking contraception (80 per cent of cases of breast cancer occur in women over the age of 50). So, compared to not taking the pill, only a small number of extra cases of breast cancer will be diagnosed. To give you the numbers, it's estimated there will be

* An extra 8 cases of breast cancer for every 100,000 women who take the pill between the ages of 16 and 20
* An extra 265 cases of breast cancer for every 100,000 women who take the pill between the ages of 35 and 39.[10]

Of course, there are some situations where it's not suitable for someone to take the pill – those with migraine with aura or high blood pressure, for example – because the risks are thought to outweigh the benefits. This is why a conversation needs to be had with a doctor (not @pill_free_Sarah_xx), so they can discuss your options in the context of your health.

Side effects aside, a lot of women tell me that they just want to 'feel themselves' or experience their natural cycle, which I think are also completely valid reasons to consider stopping the pill or not taking it in the first place. The 'right' form of contraception for you will evolve over time, and that might mean changing to a new form that suits you better now, choosing a more convenient long-term version, or taking a break from it altogether, even if it means going back on it later down the line.

What to expect when you stop taking the pill

Regardless of how long you've been taking the pill, the synthetic hormones are cleared from the body within days – and any side effects you may have experienced should subside quickly too. On the flip side, any benefits of the pill, such as lighter periods and less breakouts, that you may have experienced can disappear too, but it's very hard to predict. Most women can expect their fertility to return to their baseline within 3 cycles, but you can also get pregnant as soon as you come off the pill – so make sure you've got an alternative contraceptive method lined up if pregnancy is not something you're planning for.[11]

Although you may have a withdrawal bleed shortly after stopping the pill, this is not an actual period and typically that should return within a month, with almost all women getting their period within 3 months.[12] If it takes longer than this, you should speak to your doctor to investigate why this might be. The other thing to consider is that, since taking the pill, what's 'normal' for your body may have changed. Over that time, you may have developed a condition such as PCOS or amenorrhoea (period loss), which the pill essentially masks with a regular, monthly 'bleed' (see page XX for more on this). While some women stop taking the pill due to reports of how it impacts their mood,[13] others find it helps with PMS or PMDD (premenstrual dysphoric disorder) and therefore may notice changes in mood after stopping.

What to do before coming off hormonal contraception

* Speak with your doctor beforehand, especially if you have been using hormonal contraception to manage symptoms such as heavy or painful periods. They can also discuss alternative options for you if you would like to remain on contraception but switch the type.
* If you're planning to get pregnant, make sure to start taking folic acid for at least 3 months before conception up until the 12th week of pregnancy.
* If you wish to avoid pregnancy, consider what alternative contraception would be best for you.
* Take note of any symptoms (such as pain, heaviness, mood) and cycle length using a menstrual cycle tracking app. This will help you learn your 'new normal' and inform conversations with health professionals should any new symptoms arise.

Other types of contraception

Thankfully, since the years of the goat-bladder condom, contraception has come a long way. There are now 15 different methods of contraception available in the UK, though, that said, only 2 per cent of GPs in the UK offer all methods, and over 50 per cent of GPs feel there is not enough time in a standard appointment to discuss each of the options.[14] While this book cannot replace the medical advice your doctor can provide you with, hopefully it will help you feel more informed and educated on your options – and perhaps empowered when it comes to deciding on the right form of contraception for you.

We can categorize contraception into hormonal or non-hormonal options (figure x). They can also be divided into short-acting or user-dependent, where they need to be taken on a daily, weekly or monthly basis, such as the pill, patch, ring, and non-hormonal methods such as condoms, spermicides and the diaphragm. Forms of long-acting reversible contraception (known as LARCs) are methods where you don't need to remember to take them to be effective, and include methods like the hormonal coil, the injection, the implant, and non-hormonal methods such as the copper coil.

Non-hormonal methods

* **Condoms:** Thin sheaths worn over the penis (male condoms) or inserted into the vagina (female condoms) to prevent sperm from entering the uterus. They also prevent against sexually transmitted infections.
* **Copper IUD (intrauterine device) – 'The Coil':** The non-hormonal coil, also known as the copper coil or IUD (intrauterine device), is a small T-shaped piece of copper

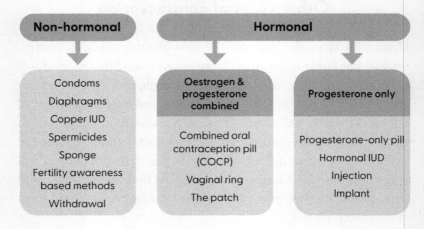

TYPES OF HORMONAL CONTRACEPTION

Non-hormonal

Condoms
Diaphragms
Copper IUD
Spermicides
Sponge
Fertility awareness
based methods
Withdrawal

Hormonal

Oestrogen & progesterone combined

Combined oral
contraception pill
(COCP)
Vaginal ring
The patch

Progesterone only

Progesterone-only pill
Hormonal IUD
Injection
Implant

and plastic that sits in the womb (uterus) and lasts for up to 10 years. It's a very effective contraceptive but it can make your periods longer and heavier.

* **Spermicide:** A chemical that kills sperm, used in forms like gels or creams, often with other forms of contraception.
* **Diaphragm:** A flexible cup inserted into the vagina to cover the cervix and used with spermicide to block sperm.
* **The sponge:** A small, soft sponge soaked in spermicide that is inserted into the vagina before sex in order to prevent pregnancy.
* **Withdrawal (pull-out method):** This involves pulling the penis out of the vagina before ejaculation to prevent sperm from entering. It's not a very reliable method of contraception (because the pre-ejaculatory fluid contains sperm), with a 1 in 5 risk of pregnancy.[15]
* **Fertility awareness-based methods (FABMs):** FABMs work by following changes in the menstrual cycle to predict ovulation and the days that sex could result in pregnancy. Traditionally, people used pen and paper to track where they were at in their cycle, but now there are over 500 menstrual

cycle tracking apps to choose from.[16] These apps use 'self-learning algorithms', meaning they work best the more a user engages and the longer the app is used. That said, period-tracking apps can get it wrong, and not all use evidence-based tracking methods (look out for versions that are FDA approved). As we learned earlier in the book, when used as a form of contraception, these methods have a high failure rate of about 1 in 3 (32 per cent), and can be as high as 1 in 2 (50 per cent) when used as the only form of contraception, with typical use.[17]

Hormonal contraception

Hormonal methods of contraception contain either oestrogen plus progesterone or progesterone and have various formulations and methods of delivery.

Oestrogen and progesterone (combined)
* **Combined oral contraceptive pill (COCP) – a.k.a. 'The Pill'**
  - Example: Yasmin, Microgynon, Rigevidon
  - Pills are typically taken daily for 21 days followed by a 7-day break or 7 days of placebo/dummy pills. Occasionally people take pill packets back to back (continuous pill taking), which is safe to do

* **Vaginal ring**
  - Example: NuvaRing
  - A flexible ring inserted into the vagina – one ring lasts 3 weeks
* **Contraceptive patch**
  - Example: Evra Patch
  - A sticky patch placed on the skin and worn for a week at a time, with a new patch each week for 3 weeks, followed by a patch-free week

Progesterone only

＊ **Progesterone-only pill (POP) – a.k.a. 'The mini pill'**
  • Example: Cerazette, Cerelle, Noriday

＊ **Hormonal intrauterine system (IUS)**
  • Example: Mirena, Jaydess
  • Small T-shaped rod inserted into the womb,
    lasts 3–5 years

＊ **Contraceptive injection**
  • Example: Depo-Provera
  • Given as an injection every 3 months

＊ **Contraceptive implant**
  • Example: Nexplanon
  • A small rod that releases progestogen, inserted under
    the skin. Lasts for 3 years but can be taken out anytime.

Choosing the right method for you involves considering a few things: convenience, potential side effects, reliability and future pregnancy plans. See the decision tree on page XXX to help you explore your options.

Hormonal contraception and its impact on the menstrual cycle

I'm often asked, 'Dr Hazel, when I'm on hormonal contraception, what happens to the hormones of my menstrual cycle?'

And the answer is . . . it depends.

Hormonal contraception can alter the natural menstrual cycle in various ways depending on the type, formulation and route of contraception.

For example, the suppression of natural oestrogen and progesterone with combined hormonal contraception options (such as the pill) means that the hormonal ups and downs that occurs with a 'normal' cycle do not happen.

Instead, it looks a little bit more like the graph below. Essentially, the pill suppresses the normal menstrual cycle and replaces it with an artificial 28-day cycle.

Diagram to follow

Source: Hirschberg A L. Challenging Aspects of Research on the Influence of the Menstrual Cycle and Oral Contraceptives on Physical Performance. *Sports Med.* 2022 Jul; 52(7): 1453-1456.[18]

* The higher levels of oestrogen and progesterone from the pills suppress the production of F S H and L H from the pituitary gland in the brain.
* Without F S H, follicle maturation doesn't occur, and without the L H surge, ovulation doesn't occur, and an egg is not released.
* When the pill-free week occurs, or placebo pills are taken, this causes a breakdown of the uterine lining, and a withdrawal bleed occurs. This is not the same as a period.

Ovulation may still occur on some progesterone-only methods of hormonal contraception, but it depends on the type, dose and route of the synthetic progesterone.[19] Just because ovulation may occur while using these methods doesn't mean that the contraception isn't working. Progesterone-only methods also work in other ways, such as thickening cervical mucus so that sperm are blocked from reaching the egg.

Finding the right form of contraception for *you*

Unfortunately, it can require a little bit of trial and error to find the right form of contraception for you, and the right choice for you can evolve over time depending on your priorities, relationship, menstrual cycle symptoms, and plans for pregnancy. This decision tree can give you an idea of what options may be suitable for you. *It goes without saying, however, that this does **not** replace a consultation with a health professional.*

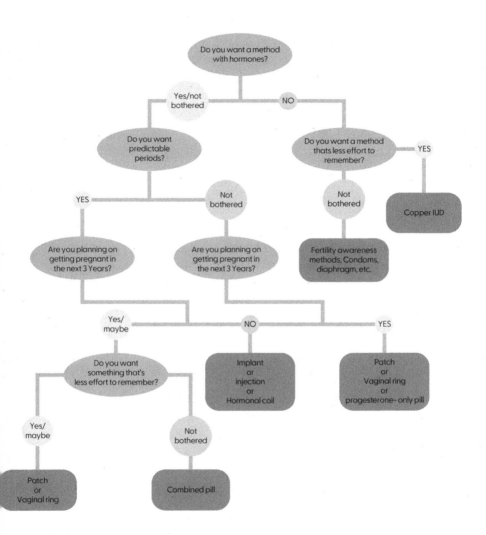

Summary

* The menstrual cycle starts on the first day of the period and ends the day before the following period begins.

* The length of menstrual cycles may vary from cycle to cycle and person to person. Between 21 and 35 days is considered normal.

* We can divide the menstrual cycle into two main phases: the follicular and luteal phase.

* Ovulation occurs on day 14 but can vary by up to 10 days.

* Hormones send signals back and forth between the brain, the ovaries and the uterus to make the cycles and their phases happen.

* Any menstrual cycle symptom causing significant disruption to daily life (i.e., work/school, social life, relationships) requires a discussion with a health professional.

* While there are legitimate concerns about the pill's side effects, social media platforms like TikTok are not reliable sources for this information; it's important to consult healthcare professionals for accurate guidance.

* Contraception options can be categorized into hormonal or non-hormonal options, with short-acting/user-dependent methods like the pill, patch, ring, condoms, spermicides and diaphragm, and long-acting reversible contraception (LARC) methods such as the hormonal coil, injection, implant, and non-hormonal copper coil.

Part 2

Living Alongside Your Cycle

By now, you should (hopefully) understand what's happening during the menstrual cycle, the hormones involved, and red-flag signs and symptoms to look out for, so that you know what to do when something isn't quite right.

What I haven't yet explained is how to optimize your health by adjusting your nutrition, movement, sleep and even your skincare across your menstrual cycle. I'm going to show you how you can take charge of your wellbeing and truly feel your best by tailoring these aspects to the different phases of your cycle. You'll discover how to navigate changes in body image, libido and mood, and how to view these elements of your health more accurately and positively through the lens of your cycle.

Our hormones have a powerful influence over our bodies, but we are not at their mercy. By understanding and working with these natural rhythms, we can harness their power, rather than constantly battling against them. This knowledge empowers you to take control of your health, make informed decisions, and embrace your cycle as a source of strength and resilience.

Nutrition

Understanding the relationship between our menstrual cycle and our diet is incredibly empowering. These two aspects of our health influence each other in powerful ways – both positively and negatively. And yet, so many women are fearful of food, constantly bombarded with messages about what to 'avoid' or 'cut out', instead of learning what to add and include in their diet and how it can truly help them.

Take it from me – I learned the hard way just how crucial nutrition and calorie intake are for a healthy cycle. In my early 20s, I lost my period after going through a weight-loss journey. While weight loss isn't inherently bad for menstrual cycle health, prolonged calorie deficits, restricting carbohydrates, and having low body fat certainly are. My 'nutrition coach' at the time reassured me it was totally normal for women to lose their period when they lose weight, so I went along with it. Reflecting on this now, I want to go back in time and shake myself for sacrificing my health in the name of thinness and beauty standards – a and for letting someone else tell me what's 'normal' for my body. It took time, regaining some weight, increasing my calorie intake and adding back the foods I'd excluded to restore my periods. Alongside these changes, a lot more joy naturally returned to my life, too.

Fast-forward a few years to my late 20s, when I was diagnosed with PCOS. Once again, food and my diet became key to managing my symptoms. Like many newly diagnosed women with

PCOS, I was advised to cut out carbohydrates, start fasting until lunchtime, and 'come back when I planned to get pregnant' – *face palm*. Fortunately, at that time, I was studying for my Masters in Clinical Nutrition and knew better than to take this consultant's nutrition 'advice' too seriously. Through evidence-backed nutrition strategies – like adding foods rich in omega-3 into my diet, choosing high-fibre carbohydrates over refined ones, and targeted supplementation – I was able to transform my cycle and improve my PCOS symptoms without cutting carbs or going on a restrictive diet.

These experiences are the reason I've dedicated my career to specializing in nutrition for women's health, and through my own practice, I'm constantly reminded how powerful nutrition is in supporting a healthy cycle and managing symptoms of menstrual-related conditions like PCOS and endometriosis.

Even if you don't have a menstrual cycle disorder, however, you can still benefit from optimizing your diet around your cycle. And no, this doesn't mean following a prescriptive meal plan for each week of your cycle, or only eating certain seeds when you're ovulating. It's about learning how to eat intuitively during different phases of your menstrual cycle. Maybe that looks like increasing the amount of colourful fruits and veggies during your period to support inflammation and uncomfortable symptoms, upping your fibre and water intake in the premenstrual phase to combat constipation and bloating, or finally getting a handle on your chocolate cravings before your period.

After all, your body's needs change throughout the menstrual cycle, and understanding this (as well as your unique needs) allows you to proactively support yourself so you feel like *you're* the one in control – not your hormones.

In this chapter, I'm going to show you how the right nutrition and tools can help you have a smoother cycle, fewer symptoms and more energy all month long.

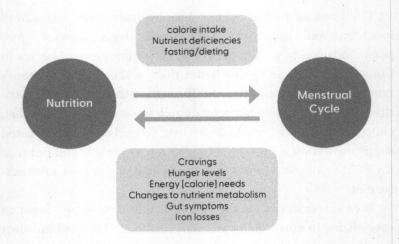

calorie intake
Nutrient deficiencies
fasting/dieting

Nutrition

Menstrual
Cycle

Cravings
Hunger levels
Energy [calorie] needs
Changes to nutrient metabolism
Gut symptoms
Iron losses

How your menstrual cycle affects your nutrition

The hormones oestrogen and progesterone not only influence our monthly cycle, but also our appetite and cravings, our metabolism, and even our gut health. All of these factors, in turn, affect how and what we eat, which influences the overall health of our cycle. In short, if we understand what our body needs and nourish it accordingly, we can support a healthier and regular menstrual cycle.

Dealing with premenstrual cravings

'Any great healthy eating habits I have or start are completely derailed the week before my period is due. I crave sugar and anything sweet. I raid the kids' sweet tin and seem to have no control over what and how much I eat. This sends me into a negative mental state about not being able to stick to my healthy eating habits.' – **Anita, 46**

One of the topics I find myself discussing with almost all my clients is dealing with premenstrual cravings and the shame and guilt that is often associated with them. It can feel almost instinctual for many women to try to restrict themselves further when they experience cravings, out of fear of losing control, or to feel bad about themselves when they succumb. The truth is, you don't have to suppress every craving, and sometimes, it's your body's way of being intuitive. I also know that feelings of guilt and shame can dissolve once you know why you're experiencing cravings.

You see, during the luteal phase of the menstrual cycle, there is a small increase in the number of calories that your body burns while at rest (known as the resting metabolic rate).[1] [2] The human body is very clever at adjusting for even small changes in metabolic rate, so during this time we also often see a natural increase in food intake and increased hunger.[3] In particular, cravings for foods high in carbohydrates and fat are very common – such as chocolate (my personal comfort food of choice). Progesterone is highest in the luteal phase, and is thought to increase appetite, whereas oestrogen may suppress it – another reason why we might observe these changes during this time. Although research is limited, some studies suggest a positive link between progesterone and binge eating, with higher levels of progesterone being associated with more frequent binge-eating episodes.[4] [5]Not all women binge-eat during hormonal fluctuations, suggesting other factors like stress might strengthen the connection between hormones and binge eating. For highly stressed women, elevated hormone levels such as oestrogen and progesterone could amplify stress responses, both mentally (feeling more stressed) and physically (higher stress hormone levels). This increased stress response can lead to more binge eating compared to women with lower stress levels.[6]

WHAT ABOUT THE PILL?

A few studies have examined how oral contraceptives impact calorie and nutrient intake, with some reporting that pill users consume more calories and fat, while others found no difference between users and non-users.[7] However, the pill may lead to an increase in binge eating in some but not *all* women – likely due to differences in genetics.[8] Regarding resting metabolic rate, results are mixed, with some studies showing an increase, others no change, and some a decrease in metabolic rate compared to non-pill users.[9]

A decrease in insulin sensitivity during the luteal phase may also play a role in cravings and how much we eat – or want to eat – during this time.[10] [11] Insulin sensitivity refers to how well your body's cells respond to insulin, allowing glucose to enter the cells and keep blood sugar levels stable. When the body is less insulin-sensitive, cells don't take up glucose easily, leading to higher insulin production. This shift is thought to occur to help store energy and build fat for a potential pregnancy. However, some studies have reported no changes in insulin sensitivity, so it is likely to be very individual and dependent on associated factors such as high BMI, low cardiorespiratory fitness levels and conditions associated with insulin resistance such as PCOS.[12]

While these changes may be hormonally driven, we can make informed choices to help manage our cravings and energy levels and prevent a binge:

* Aim to have regular, balanced meals that include high-fibre carbohydrates (think brown rice, wholemeal bread and wholegrains) paired with protein and healthy fats to help stabilize blood sugar and energy levels, and to make the meal more satisfying and filling. This isn't a strict

rule that you have to follow, but a guide that can be used flexibly.

* Avoid skipping meals or pushing your meals back by a few hours in an attempt to curb calorie intake, as this can backfire and lead to overeating later in the day.

* Once we have considered our physical hunger needs, we should then investigate our emotional needs – we all have them, and that's a good thing (it's what makes us human!). Sometimes, when we perceive the urge to eat despite a lack of physical hunger, what we are really hungry for is a sense of connection, belonging, soothing or something else entirely.

* Understand that it's okay to comfort eat sometimes and give yourself permission to have what you are craving. While food is indeed fuel – food is an emotional activity at its core. Making a comforting family recipe because you're feeling homesick or lonely, meeting a mate for a catchup over cake to discuss dating dilemmas, or eating some chocolate for pure enjoyment can all be forms of self-care that make you feel better and less likely to binge than if you restricted yourself. *The problem arises when food becomes the primary, if not the only, coping strategy for managing our feelings.*

* If you do struggle with overeating, avoid eating straight out of large containers, like ice cream tubs or crisp bags. Instead, serve yourself a reasonable amount in a bowl and put the rest away. Seconds don't have to be off-limits, but the key is that you're making an intentional choice to have more and are not mindlessly eating out of boredom or stress.

* Binge-eating episodes, when you have eaten an uncomfortable amount of food in a way that feels out of control, can be really challenging and distressing. So, if they do happen, try to avoid further restriction, beating yourself

up about it, compensatory methods, body checking or isolating yourself.

✳ Movement and sleep can also make the body more insulin-sensitive – another reason to get more of them during this time.

✳ Stress can interfere with insulin's ability to regulate blood sugar levels, so it's important to prioritize relaxation and to have tools to reduce stress.

If you struggle with binge eating and don't currently have support with this, it is really important to seek this out, as getting the right support in place as soon as possible is vital for recovery and healing your relationship with food.

How your body uses fuel changes across the menstrual cycle

Whether you exercise competitively, doing marathons or triathlons, casually with a weekly Park Run or Pilates on the weekend – or even if your activity is just the daily hustle of work, household chores or chasing after the kids – it's important to know how your body's energy needs change throughout your menstrual cycle and what this means for you.

The hormones oestrogen and progesterone play a big role in how your body manages energy, even if you're not hitting the gym daily.

Carbs and fat are the main energy sources we use during activity or exercise. For example, when you're doing something more intense, like running or a boot camp session, your body relies more on carbs stored in your muscles. On the other hand, for lower-intensity activities – like walking, light yoga, or even everyday tasks – your body tends to burn more fat for fuel.

Interestingly, women tend to burn more fat than men at the same intensity level.[13] [14] [15] [16] [17] This means that even when doing moderate-intensity activities, your body might be using more fat and less carbohydrate for energy. That's not to say carbs are not still incredibly important during this time, especially for high-intensity performance, but sparing the carbohydrate stores can help women avoid 'hitting the wall', allowing them to keep going longer and, theoretically, making them well-suited for endurance sports like long-distance running, cycling and swimming.

Even though you might not be training for a marathon, understanding how your hormones affect energy use can still be useful. For example, oestrogen helps your body break down fat and use it efficiently as fuel.[18] Progesterone supports oestrogen's effort to save carbs, so when both hormones are high in the luteal phase, women tend to rely less on carbohydrates for fuel compared to those in the follicular phase, during moderate-intensity endurance exercise.[19] [20] In addition to burning more fat for fuel in the luteal phase, there is also increased use and breakdown of protein – which also comes with increased metabolic rate during this time.[21] [22] [23] This might mean women would benefit from increasing their intake of healthy fats (like fish, olive oil and avocado) and protein (from meat, fish or beans).

It's worth saying that the research is mixed on this subject, and some studies show differences in how women use fuel across the menstrual cycle, while others don't find much variation. So, while there are sports nutrition guidelines that suggest tweaking your diet based on your cycle – like eating more protein and healthy fats in the luteal phase, and more carbs in the follicular phase – it's not a one-size-fits-all approach. The way your body's hormones affect the food you eat isn't the same as the way someone else's does, so, if you're curious, experiment with these strategies to see if they help you feel more energized during your everyday activities or casual exercise sessions. It's all about finding what works best for your body and your lifestyle.

Gut changes across the menstrual cycle

Most women are comfortable talking about the cramps, bloating, skin changes and mood changes that they experience around the time of their period, but not many are talking about their period poo. I know, you know what I mean.

Even though no one really talks about it, gut symptoms, such as bloating and diarrhoea, are so incredibly common around the time of menstruation. In a group of 156 healthy women, with no history of gut disorders, nearly three-quarters of the group experienced at least one major gut symptom just before their period and two-thirds during their period.[24] The most common symptoms were abdominal (tummy) pain and diarrhoea, but constipation and bloating are also common (table x). For women with an underlying gut condition like irritable bowel syndrome (IBS), symptoms typically flare up just before and during menstruation.[25] [26]

Proportion of women experiencing gastrointestinal symptoms, comparing prevalence rates in premenstrual and menstruation

Symptoms	Pre-menstrual	During menses
Primary gastrointestinal (GI) symptoms	%	%
Abdominal pain	58	55
Diarrhoea	24	28
Nausea	17	14
Constipation	15	10
Vomiting	2	3
Any primary symptoms	73	69

Multiple (≥2) primary symptoms	31	31
Secondary GI symptoms		
Bloating	62	51
Pelvic pain	49	46
Any primary or secondary GI symptoms	83	83

Adapted from: 'Gastrointestinal symptoms before and during menses in healthy women' by M. T. Bernstein et al., 2013, *BMC Women's Health*, 14:14 (doi: 10.1186/1472-6874-14-14).[27]

These changes in gut function and uncomfortable symptoms are thought to be due to the varying levels of oestrogen and progesterone throughout the menstrual cycle. Clinical studies show that both hormones influence how the gut moves and how easily substances pass through the gut wall by acting on receptors in the digestive system.[28] For example, if you notice that you typically become more constipated before your period, this is because progesterone slows down the speed of our gut. Then, as progesterone levels drop as the next cycle begins, and your period starts, you might experience the opposite problem. Inflammatory prostaglandins, which cause the uterus to contract and shed during the period, also affect the nearby gut, leading to reduced absorption and increased secretion of water and salts, all of which can cause pain and loose stools (hello, period poops).[29]

Oestrogen is also known to affect how sensitive the gut is, which is a key feature of irritable bowel syndrome (IBS). This is thought to be a contributing factor as to why IBS is twice as common in women compared to men.[30]

Recently, it was found that oestrogen can also influence the diversity and makeup of the gut microbiome (the trillions of bacteria and other microbes that live in your gut). The relationship appears to go both ways, as there are certain gut bugs that are involved in oestrogen metabolism.[31] [32] This interaction has led researchers to believe that disruptions in the microbiome may affect how oestrogen is processed in the body and may play a role in women's health conditions such as endometriosis and PCOS.[33] More research is needed here, but looking after your gut is likely to have positive effects on your menstrual cycle and overall health.

Strategies to relieve period-related gut symptoms

* Tracking your symptoms around your cycle is always a smart way to start. I recommend doing this for at least 3 cycles – that way, you can see if there is a pattern with your gut symptoms and your cycle. If you suspect that you may be more sensitive to certain foods at this time, you could also temporarily track your food intake alongside this to see if there are any patterns.
* A lot of the advice that we went through when it comes to reducing the risk of binge eating can also help with relieving gut symptoms, e.g. eating regularly, not skipping meals and prioritizing movement, rest and relaxation (see page xx).
* Caffeine, alcohol, spicy foods, fatty/greasy foods and fizzy drinks may worsen symptoms, so best to reduce them just before and during your period.
* Try to eat slowly and chew your food well.
* Peppermint oil capsules may relieve abdominal cramping and bloating, particularly if you have irritable bowel syndrome (IBS).
* If you're really suffering from bloating, flatulence or diarrhoea, you may wish to reduce your portion sizes of foods such as beans and lentils and cruciferous vegetables (such as broccoli, cauliflower and sprouts), and avoid food or drinks that contain the sweeteners sorbitol, mannitol or xylitol for a couple of days. You could also seek support

from a gut-specialist dietitian to help with pinpointing your potential triggers.

* Similarly, if you know you always experience constipation at a particular time of the month, you may want to increase your fluid and fibre intake and consider adding flaxseed (gradually) to your daily diet.

* Don't forget, the gut and brain are very much interlinked, and women who experience depressive and anxiety symptoms are more likely to report multiple gut symptoms.[34] The days leading up to, and during, your period is an ideal time to include some stress-relieving activities such as meditation, yoga, breathwork or even a simple bubble bath.

How nutrition can support your cycle

Just as our menstrual cycle affects our cravings, nutrient and energy needs, and gut health, our diet can also impact menstrual health. For instance, women with low levels of certain nutrients are more likely to experience painful periods and PMS. Additionally, consuming too few calories can disrupt hormonal signals, leading to irregular or missed periods. The good news is that knowing this, and what nutrients are important at particular times in your cycle, can lead to less symptoms and improved energy overall.

A healthy menstrual cycle needs calories

In a world of fad diets and restrictive eating plans, the term 'calorie' has become a dirty word. It's often spoken about as something to be avoided or limited, but here's the deal: Your body needs calories to perform basic biological functions. Your body needs calories to do basic things like keeping your immune system working, thinking clearly, and having regular periods.

Too few calories or too little of any macronutrient (i.e., carbs/

fats/protein) can switch off the communication between the brain (hypothalamus) and the ovaries, leading to irregular or absent periods. This is the body's way of saying, 'We are not safe to make a baby right now,' and instead prioritizes energy towards more important, life-sustaining functions, like keeping the heart pumping. Think of it like the power-saving mode on a mobile phone – it extends your battery by reducing non-essential functions.

This situation is known as low energy deficiency (LEA), and happens when your body doesn't have enough energy left for important health-sustaining functions after you account for the energy you used for physical activity.

LEA underpins hypothalamic amenorrhoea (HA) and relative energy deficiency in sport (RED-S; see page XXX), and can lead to a host of symptoms (see box below).

RED-FLAG SIGNS AND SYMPTOMS THAT YOUR BODY IS LOW ON ENERGY

* Absent or irregular menstrual cycles
* Constant fatigue
* Recurrent illness or infection
* Inability to gain muscle or build strength
* Poor performance (or a plateau in performance)
* Stress fractures or bone injuries
* Gut symptoms
* Weight loss
* Low libido
* Low mood and depression

LEA can be caused by an imbalance in energy, created by a high level of exercise, a decreased food intake, or both. This can happen intentionally, for example, if you started a diet with the intention of losing weight, or unintentionally, perhaps if you started training

Diagram to follow

From: Arroyo F, Benardot D, Hernandez E. Within-day energy
balance in Mexican female soccer (football) players-an exploratory
investigation. *Int. J. Sports Exerc. Med.* 2018;4:107.[36]

for a marathon and misjudged how many extra calories your body
would need.

In addition to meeting your calorie needs, meal timing and the
distribution of calories across the day matters too. For example,
if there are big gaps in the day where enough calories aren't consumed, we risk creating a 'within-day deficit'. In other words, even
though there might be energy balance by the end of the day, if very
large chunks of the day are spent in negative energy balance, your
body will start making metabolic adjustments to account for it.
Small, infrequent deficits are unlikely to be harmful, but when your
energy falls below -300kcal, this seems to be the threshold for when
negative consequences arise.[35]

Practically speaking, then, let's take a look at these scenarios:

Scenario A

﹡ You wake up at 6 a.m. and head to the gym before eating (you
might have a black coffee, but that's it). You are already in an

energy deficit because not only did you not eat, but you are using more energy to exercise.

* After the gym, you shower, get ready for work, and squeeze in a quick breakfast at the office on your 11am break.
* By lunchtime, you're still full from breakfast so have a small snack and a coffee to tide you over.
* Your next meal is dinner, and you are *ravenous*. You quickly make dinner (grazing while you cook) and then follow up with some sweet snacks because the meal wasn't that satisfying.
* Or, for a similar story for those of you with kids, let's look at another scenario:

Scenario B

* You're woken up at 6am by your four-year-old and seven-year-old, and get up straight away to make them breakfast. You immediately have a black coffee for energy. You don't eat yourself, as you don't have time to prepare yourself something alongside the two different meals that they both want, before leaving the house to take them to nursery and school.
* You drop your four-year-old at nursery and seven-year-old at school, a round trip of 2 miles by foot, then hotfoot it to the bus to catch it to the tube for work.
* Once at work, you're straight into meetings, so only have time to grab a cereal bar or a banana.
* Your only chance to exercise is at lunch, where you manage to run a 5k and use the office showers before your afternoon starts. You're absolutely starving by now, so you grab a lacklustre sandwich from the high street and a few biscuits from the office kitchen to keep you going for the afternoon.

* You're still hungry when you're making dinner for the kids, so you graze while cooking for them, and also finish their leftovers, as well as eating your own meal. You follow up with some sweet snacks once the kids are in bed.

In both of these situations, even if you're getting enough energy by the end of the day, chances are your body is still experiencing physical stress and its repercussions during the times you're fasting. This is one of the reasons why I personally don't advocate for fasted exercise in women, as it dramatically pushes the energy balance into negative territory. Fasting in general can also make it difficult to get enough energy and nutrients across the day, and can worsen disordered eating behaviours.[37]

Now take a look at these alternative scenarios:

Scenario C

* You wake up at 6am, still drink your morning coffee, but this time you have a banana before the gym and pack your prepped overnight oats.
* You shower and change after the gym, but as you've brought your breakfast with you, you have time to eat before work starts at 9am.
* By lunchtime, you're sufficiently hungry but not ravenous, and choose a balanced lunch with protein, carbs and fats.
* You have an afternoon pot of yoghurt and some fruit at 3pm.
* By the time you get around to making dinner at 7pm, you're not feeling rushed or ravenous and take your time to make a satisfying meal that doesn't leave you hungry. You have a couple of squares of dark chocolate and feel comfortably full and satisfied going to bed.

Or, for those trying to balance looking after your body with looking after your children:

Scenario D

* You're woken at 6am by your four-year-old and seven-year-old, and get up straight away to make them breakfast. You still need/want that morning caffeine hit, so you still drink your coffee, but last night you prepped some overnight oats, or ensured that you had some wholewheat bread to make an easy slice of toast or two, so eat while tending to the kids. You grab a banana to take to the office.
* You drop your four-year-old at nursery and seven-year-old at school, a round trip of 2 miles by foot, then hotfoot it to the bus to catch it to the tube for work.
* Once at work, you're straight into meetings, but you have your banana at your 11 am break, which tops up your energy stores ahead of your lunchtime run.
* In your lunch break, you run a 5k and use the office showers before your afternoon starts. You grab a sandwich, as well as some fruit and nuts to snack on in the afternoon. By the time the 4pm tea time comes round, you don't need biscuits for energy.
* Because you've had a balanced lunch, when you're home and making dinner for the kids, you don't feel the need to graze and you can manage your own portion size rather than adding their leftovers to your own plate.

In these situations, even if you consumed the same amount of calories as you did in the previous scenarios, you haven't spent chunks of the day in an energy deficit. Your body feels **safe**, **fuelled** and **nourished**.

If you're actively pursuing weight loss, you might wonder how to navigate this while in a deficit. Regardless of your body size, you're still at risk of menstrual disturbances on a weight-loss journey, but you can help mitigate the risk by avoiding fasting, skipping meals or 'saving calories' for later in the day. You can still achieve your weight-loss goals by eating regular, balanced meals and maintaining a mild but sustainable energy deficit.

Body weight and the menstrual cycle

We've explored how having a very low body weight or going through a weight-loss journey can negatively affect your menstrual cycle, causing it to become irregular or disappear. However, excess body weight can also have the potential to negatively affect the menstrual cycle, leading to irregular cycles, heavier periods, as well as having an impact on fertility.

A NOTE ON BODY MASS INDEX (BMI)

Before we jump into it, I want to briefly discuss BMI, or body mass index, so that we're all on the same page.

BMI is a screening tool used to determine if someone has a 'healthy' weight relative to their height. It categorizes individuals into underweight (below a BMI of 18.5), healthy weight (18.5 to 24.9), overweight (25 to 29.9) and obese (>30). For those with Asian, Chinese, Middle Eastern, Black African or African-Caribbean family background, a lower BMI score is used to measure overweight (23 to 27.4) and obese (>27.5).

Despite its common use, BMI has a number of limitations. For one, it doesn't distinguish between muscle and fat, so a person with a lot of muscle mass (such as a weight lifter or rugby player) might be classified as overweight or obese despite being incredibly fit and healthy. BMI also doesn't tell us where that fat is distributed, which is important, because fat around the abdomen (tummy area) poses a higher risk to health than fat carried in the bottom and thighs. BMI also doesn't factor in diet, physical activity levels and metabolic health (such as cholesterol and glucose levels) – all of which influence health and our risk of disease. So, when I discuss BMI, or body weight, in clinic, I always highlight these limitations and emphasize the importance of not looking at the number on the scales (or BMI) in isolation, without interpreting it alongside other health markers – such as menstrual cycle regularity.

Having a higher body weight can increase the risk of a number of menstrual cycle issues.

Heavy periods

Obesity is a risk factor for heavy periods likely due to inflammation, reduced ability for the womb lining to heal, and changes in hormone levels as a result of excess body fat.[1] Adipose (fat) tissue produces oestrogen, so having excess fat can increase oestrogen levels in the body. Higher oestrogen can make the womb's lining grow thicker and have more blood vessels, leading to heavier periods. In addition, obesity is a risk factor for cancer of the womb, which can sometimes cause heavy bleeding.

Irregular cycles

Studies have found that people with a higher body weight are more likely to experience irregular cycles.[2] [3] This may be because a higher fat mass is associated with insulin resistance, a condition where the body's cells don't respond effectively to insulin, and this then sets off a chain of events. Elevated insulin levels can stimulate the ovaries to produce more androgens (male hormones), such as testosterone. High androgen levels can interfere with the development of ovarian follicles and ovulation, leading to irregular or absent menstrual cycles. Inflammation and higher oestrogen levels, as a result of excess adipose tissue, can also contribute to irregular cycles.

PCOS

While having a higher body weight does not cause PCOS (and women of all shapes and sizes can have it), having a higher body weight can worsen the condition by contributing to insulin resistance and therefore driving up levels of sex hormones. In women with PCOS who have a higher body weight, weight loss (of 5–10 per cent) can help with symptoms, including regulating periods and improving fertility.[4] But it's important to say that PCOS can make losing weight harder, and women with PCOS already have a higher risk of disordered eating and body image issues, so weight loss isn't always a helpful focus.[5]

Fibroids

A high BMI has also been linked to an increased risk of uterine fibroids (which are non-cancerous growths that develop in or around the uterus), possibly due to excess oestrogen produced from fat tissue and increased inflammation.[6] Many women are unaware they have fibroids because they do not have any symptoms, but for those that do, heavy or painful periods are the most common. (See page xx for more on fibroids.)

Fertility

Having too little or too much body fat can also potentially impact fertility.

One study, that is often cited, surveyed 2,112 pregnant women and found:[7]

* Women with BMIs under 19 took, on average, 29 months to conceive.
* Women with BMIs between 19 and 24 took, on average, 6.8 months to conceive.
* Women with BMIs between 25 and 39 took, on average, 10.6 months to conceive.
* Women with BMIs above 39 took, on average, 13.3 months to conceive.

The study's findings remained the same after accounting for other lifestyle variables (like smoking and caffeine and alcohol intake), menstrual cycle regularity and age. Based on data like this, healthcare professionals may recommend weight gain or loss for people with fertility issues and BMIs outside the 'average' range. This isn't easy for everyone, however, and some people may need support from their doctor, a therapist and/or a dietitian/nutritionist to make significant changes to their relationship with eating and exercise.

There is also a lot of weight stigma in health and healthcare and that includes women's health. Unfortunately, women with higher body weight often have their menstrual issues blamed on their weight without looking into other possible causes. Studies show women with a high BMI get fewer cervical cancer screenings and have less access to fertility treatments because of weight bias.[8] [9] [10] Having a weight loss target as a barrier to fertility treatment can be extremely difficult, as this can add more stress at a time when most people are already feeling vulnerable, especially if you have struggled with your weight, body image or relationship with food in the past. While it is sometimes necessary for your doctor to discuss your weight when it comes to your health, other factors must be taken into consideration too. If you feel comfortable, you can explain to your doctor or nurse that you'd like to be treated holistically – beyond your BMI or a number on the scale. If routine weigh-ins are part of your care, you can also request not to see or discuss the number if you find it triggering.

Case Study: Mia

Mia, a 21-year-old student, experienced amenorrhea (loss of periods) for 7 months. After a health assessment with her medical team, she was initially told that her period loss was due to a high BMI and was advised to lose weight. Mia then reached out to me for nutrition support, and upon reviewing her previous blood tests, I noticed high testosterone and low sex hormone-binding globulin (SHBG) levels, consistent with PCOS. I recommended she get a second opinion, which led to her receiving a diagnosis of PCOS. Her gynaecologist prescribed medication to help manage her condition, and I provided nutritional support to help with her symptoms. We implemented a regular eating schedule and a low glycaemic index (GI) diet, along with targeted supplementation, to manage PCOS, while also focusing on improving sleep, increasing physical activity and managing stress (see page xx for more on PCOS and diet).

This case highlights the importance of a thorough assessment for women with irregular or absent periods, especially in larger bodies, rather than attributing symptoms solely to body weight. While weight loss can be beneficial for some women with PCOS (and a high BMI), in Mia's case, without having a diagnosis of PCOS, she wouldn't have had access to medication to support her health condition, and she wouldn't have received the appropriate nutrition and lifestyle advice from me.

Nutrition can help ease menstrual symptoms

You might stumble across recipes or claims about foods that 'ease' period pain while scrolling through social media, and while one food is unlikely to cure cramps, certain nutrients have been found to reduce the likelihood of painful periods. Menstruation, in and of itself, is an inflammatory process, and high levels of inflammatory markers in the bloodstream have been linked to menstrual symptom severity and PMS.[11] The nutrients listed below, such as omega-3 fatty acids, magnesium and zinc, are known to have anti-inflammatory and antioxidant properties and have been shown to help ease symptoms associated with menstruation.[12] Include them in your diet where possible, and if you're considering taking supplements to top up your stores, make sure to chat to your pharmacist or doctor first.

Omega-3 fatty acids

Omega-3 fatty acids can reduce the production of inflammatory prostaglandins that drive pain during menstruation. Studies have shown that women who take a daily omega-3 supplement experience less pain and require fewer doses of anti-inflammatory painkillers (such as ibuprofen) to manage pain.[13] [14]

Omega-3 fatty acids are a type of polyunsaturated fatty acids and are considered essential, meaning that we must obtain them through our diet or through supplements, as our body cannot create them. The active forms of omega-3, docosahexaenoic acid (DHA) and eicosapentaenoic acid (EPA), are found mainly in oily fish. These are also present in seaweed and algae. Another form of omega-3, alpha-linolenic acid (ALA), is found in plant-based foods like flax and chia seeds, walnuts, rapeseed and soybean oil, and soya-based foods. However, only a small amount of ALA is converted into EPA and DHA. Therefore, a supplement is generally advisable for those who don't consume oily fish.

From the research, there doesn't seem to be an agreed-upon effective dose for reducing menstrual pain, but most studies use a 1000mg fish/marine oil supplement with 300mg omega-3 (180mg EPA and 120mg DHA).[15] For general health, the UK government recommends adults take 450mg of combined EPA and DHA per day, which works out as around the same as a 140g portion of oily fish per week.[16] [17] Oily fish include salmon, herring, sardines, pilchards, trout, mackerel and sprats. Fresh and canned tuna no longer count as oily fish, as they don't contain the high levels of polyunsaturated fats of other oily fish.

SMASH is a handy acronym to help you remember five cold-water fish with good amounts of omega-3 fatty acids : salmon, mackerel, anchovies, sardines and herring.

Calcium

Calcium plays a role in muscle contraction, and low levels can lead to an increase in cramping of the uterus, which can cause pain. Calcium supplementation alone, or in combination with magnesium, has been shown to relieve menstrual pain. In these studies, supplementation was taken from day 15 of the cycle until pain disappeared the following cycle.[18] [19] As a starting point, I would aim to include 3–4 servings of dairy (or calcium-fortified alternatives) per day. Other sources include green leafy vegetables, tahini, calcium-set tofu, dried figs, nuts and seeds, and tinned fish with bones.

Vitamin D

Vitamin D is important for increasing calcium absorption from the gut and also plays a large role in regulating inflammation. Some studies have shown that the severity of painful periods increases with decreasing vitamin D levels in the blood, and supplementation has been shown to reduce the severity of pain.[20] However, not all studies have found an improvement.[21] That said, regardless of whether you experience menstrual pain or not, the UK government recommended that all adults take a 10mcg supplement of vitamin D during autumn and winter, as it is difficult to obtain enough from our diet. While most of our vitamin D is made through our skin when we are outside in sunlight, it can also be found in egg yolks, oily fish, liver and fortified foods.

Magnesium

Magnesium helps the uterus muscles relax and reduces the production of pain-inducing prostaglandins. It's been found that magnesium levels in women with painful periods is also typically low, compared to those without, and trials where supplementation has been used seem to be effective in reducing the severity of pain.[22][23] We don't yet know the best dose or schedule for taking magnesium to treat period pain because the studies vary too much, with some using daily doses, and others initiating treatment in the luteal phase.[24][25][26] So, more research is needed before we can make a solid recommendation, but you might like to try including more magnesium-rich foods and seeing if that works for you. Magnesium can be found in pumpkin seeds, nuts, spinach, black beans, soya beans, whole grains and dark chocolate.

Note: Magnesium supplements can cause diarrhoea (especially at doses >400mg) and also interact or interfere with some medicines and compete for absorption with other minerals like iron and zinc. It's always best to consult your doctor or pharmacist before starting any new supplements.

Zinc

Zinc is an essential mineral involved in immune function, wound healing, DNA synthesis and numerous other bodily processes. Limited research suggests that zinc might be helpful in reducing period pain when taken around menstruation.[27] [28] [29]This could be due to several reasons, such as improving blood flow and preventing tissue damage, neutralizing harmful molecules and reducing inflammation. Zinc may also reduce the production of pain-causing compounds in a way similar to anti-inflammatory drugs like NSAIDs. In fact, when used in combination with the non-steroidal anti-inflammatory medication mefenamic acid, it has been shown to be more effective at reducing painful periods compared to mefenamic acid alone.[30] Zinc can be found in many foods, including meat, dairy (especially cheese), shellfish, nuts and seeds, wholegrains, beans, chickpeas and lentils.

Note: As with magnesium, high doses of zinc can block absorption of other minerals. Too much zinc can also lead to temporary gut issues and vomiting.[31]

Curcumin (turmeric)

Curcumin is a compound in the spice turmeric and is pretty well known for its anti-inflammatory and antioxidant properties. A few studies[32] [33] [34] [35] have found supplementation with curcumin can help to alleviate symptoms of painful periods and PMS. Similar to zinc, when combined with the anti-inflammatory painkiller mefenamic acid, it is more effective than mefenamic acid alone.[36] In these studies, participants were asked to take the supplement in the days just before their next period until just after the period ended. One of curcumin's greatest disadvantages is that it is poorly absorbed when orally ingested by itself, but adding black pepper has been seen to increase its bioavailability (i.e., its absorption and function in the body) by 2000 per cent.[37]

DOES THE PILL DEPLETE NUTRIENTS?

Research has found that women on oral contraceptives, compared to those who are not, may have lower levels of the nutrients folic acid, certain B vitamins, vitamin C and E and the minerals magnesium, selenium and zinc.[38] It is unclear how the pill depletes nutrients, but it may be due to reduced absorption, increased metabolism, or excretion of these nutrients.

There are a number of cautions and limitations with the research, however.

* Most of the studies were conducted in the 1970s and 80s, with a very small handful from the early 2000s, and most have very small sample sizes.

* Some of the studies acknowledge, or have shown, that with adequate dietary intake, the risk of deficiency is low.[39]

* Essentially, all studies are based on women taking oral contraceptive pills (of various formulations). In fact, one study that did look at the pill and the injection reported a significant increase in the nutrients calcium, magnesium and phosphorus with the injection.[40]

So, before anyone panics, we need more up-to-date research on all forms of hormonal contraception to better understand this risk, so we can better inform women. With that said, anyone who is prescribed the pill should be made aware of these potential risks so that they can proactively optimize their nutrition, and for those who are already at risk of nutritional deficiencies, careful monitoring, and potentially supplementation, may be required.

* **Vitamin B2:** Dairy, eggs, mushrooms, wholegrains, meat and liver,* seafood, fortified drinks and breakfast cereals.

* **Vitamin B6:** Certain fortified cereals, oats, dairy, meat, liver,* tuna, nuts and seeds.

* **Vitamin B12:** Meat, seafood, dairy, eggs, turkey, and fortified products including nutritional yeast, certain cereals and drinks.

* **Folate:** Green vegetables like kale, cabbage, broccoli, Brussels' sprouts, lettuce and spinach, beans and peas, liver* and fortified cereals.

* **Vitamin C:** Citrus fruits, bell peppers, tomatoes, sweet potatoes and green leafy veg.

* **Vitamin E:** Olive oil, nuts and seeds, wheat germ and wholegrains.

* **Magnesium:** Nuts and seeds, spinach, black beans, soya beans and dark chocolate.

* **Selenium:** Nuts (especially Brazil nuts!), seeds, meat, fish, eggs, beans and pulses.

* **Zinc:** Meat, dairy (especially cheese), shellfish, beans and chickpeas, nuts and seeds, and quinoa.

---

* Liver and liver products such as liver pâté are a particularly rich source of vitamin A, so it is advisable not to have them more than once a week, as excess vitamin A in the form of retinol can lead to stomach pain, nausea, vomiting, irritability, headaches, skin issues and liver damage. A high intake of vitamin A can harm an unborn baby, so pregnant women or those planning a pregnancy are advised to avoid supplements containing vitamin A, liver and liver-containing products like pâté.

Nutrition for each phase

Bringing this all together, you might be thinking about how you should eat for each phase of your cycle, but I would caution that it's a little too early to say. Research in this field is in its infancy (and conflicting), so we don't have enough evidence yet to start making blanket recommendations for *all* women. I personally don't recommend rigid meal plans or food rules to my clients when it comes to their menstrual cycle (or any other health goal), so the advice provided here should be used as a flexible guide, not the rule.

Menstrual cycle phase	Hormones	Impact on nutrition and food intake	Potential diet tweaks
Menstruation (the start to the end of the period)	Oestrogen and progesterone are low	Inflammation, iron losses and gut symptoms	⬆ Anti-inflammatory foods (think colourful fruit and vegetables, oily fish, nuts and seeds) ⬆ Iron-rich foods (red meat, fortified cereals, eggs, beans, lentils and chickpeas, tofu, green leafy veg, nuts and seeds, dried fruit) ⬆ Pair plant-based foods containing iron with foods rich in vitamin C rich (think citrus fruits, peppers, leafy greens and tomatoes) to increase iron absorption. Avoid coffee and tea at meal times, which can impair iron absorption. ✗ Caution with foods and drinks that stimulate the gut: coffee, alcohol, fatty and spicy meals, sugar-free foods.
Late follicular phase (after the period to ovulation)	Oestrogen rises, progesterone remains low	Insulin sensitivity ⬆ Appetite and cravings ➡	↺ Continue to follow a healthy, balanced diet with healthy fats, adequate protein and complex carbohydrates. ⬆ Focus on gut health with probiotic foods, such as kefir and yoghurts, with live active cultures, and prebiotics such as artichokes, onion, garlic, asparagus and leeks.

Menstrual cycle phase	Hormones	Impact on nutrition and food intake	Potential diet tweaks
Luteal phase (from ovulation to the next period)	Progesterone and oestrogen peak mid-luteal phase	⬆ Increase in metabolic rate, cravings and hunger ⬇ Insulin sensitivity ⬆ Risk of constipation	⬆ Complex carbohydrates, protein and healthy fats at each meal (eating regularly – not skipping meals). ⬆ Increase high-fibre foods from wholegrains, fruit and veg, and flaxseed to support constipation (if an issue). ❤ Give yourself permission to eat foods that you are craving, and also try to meet your overall emotional needs. ⬆ Increase foods rich in omega-3, calcium, magnesium and zinc to support PMS and menstrual cramps (continue throughout menstruation). Consider supplementation if needed.

Summary

* The menstrual cycle, and the hormones oestrogen and progesterone, influence cravings, hunger levels, energy and nutrient needs, and gut function.

* Similarly, our nutrition and dietary habits can influence our menstrual cycle health, including pain, PMS and regularity.

* During the luteal phase, there is a potential increase in resting metabolic rate. Women typically report higher cravings, hunger levels and increased food intake during this time.

* Gut symptoms, such as bloating and diarrhoea, are common before and during menstruation.

* Adequate calorie intake is crucial for a healthy menstrual cycle. Low energy availability can lead to menstrual disturbances and other health issues.

* Having a higher body weight can lead to menstrual issues like heavier or irregular periods. It may also increase the risk of fibroids and fertility challenges.

* Certain nutrients like omega-3 fatty acids, calcium, vitamin D, magnesium and zinc can help reduce menstrual pain and inflammation.

Movement

Women's participation in sport and exercise has a long, complex history filled with both challenges and triumphs. Back in the late 19th century, many male doctors believed that women were physically and mentally limited by their menstrual cycles.[1] Harvard Professor Dr Edward Clarke even claimed women needed to rest both their bodies and brains during their periods, due to the rationale that any exertion would sap energy from their reproductive systems.[2]

But not everyone agreed. In 1874, Dr Mary Putnam Jacobi challenged Clarke's ideas with a scientific study on 268 menstruating women, measuring various physical capabilities throughout their cycles.[3] She concluded in her paper titled 'The Question of Rest for Women during Menstruation' that there was no evidence to suggest women need to rest during their periods, once they are nourished and healthy.[4] Not only did Jacobi's study debunk Clarke's claim, it also won her an award: the Boylston Medical Prize at Harvard – the same school where Clarke taught.

Even as scientific evidence started to show that periods don't hinder physical performance, these outdated views persisted into the 20th century. For example, the International Olympic Committee once believed that sports training and competition could harm women's reproductive health. It was believed that anything over an 800m run was dangerous to female fertility – with some claiming it would cause a woman's womb to fall out![5] [6] When Roberta 'Bobbi' Gibb applied to run the 1966 Boston Marathon, organisers told her,

'Women are not physiologically capable of running a marathon.'[7] Bobbi proved them wrong by sneaking into the race and becoming the first woman to run it.

It wasn't until 1972 that women were *finally* allowed to run the New York City Marathon, but even then, they had to start 10 minutes before the men. The six women entered in the race protested by sitting down at the starting line and only starting when the men did.[8]

Since then, women have continued to break barriers in sports. The Paris 2024 Olympics was the first sex-equal Games, with an equal number of spots for male and female athletes. However, women and girls still lag behind men in physical activity levels.[9] Cultural norms, safety concerns, body image issues, limited opportunity and menstrual cycle-related concerns all contribute to this disparity.[10][11][12][13]

A 2023 survey revealed that over 80 per cent of teenage girls lost interest in sports after starting their menstrual cycle, and nearly 1 in 4 say they feel embarrassed to exercise during their period.[14] As a former teenage girl, and (former) keen football player, I understand this anxiety. I vividly remember getting my period during a game, unknowingly, while wearing an all-white kit and getting benched by the coach without any explanation (although the sniggers and pointing from the sidelines soon made it clear). The shame and embarrassment of that moment made me so fearful of participating in sports during my period, and it took me a long time to get over.

Small changes like offering the choice to wear non-white sports kits or coloured undershorts, should girls and women feel more comfortable to, can go a long way. That, at last, seems to be happening, as England and Ireland women's rugby teams have changed out of white shorts, and Wimbledon now allows female tennis players to wear coloured undershorts.[15][16]

Of course, clothing isn't the only barrier. Between 36 per cent and 93 per cent of active women believe their menstrual cycle or hormonal contraceptive influences their ability to perform in sports and exercise.[17] [18] Menstrual symptoms can affect not just how well we do in sport and exercise, but also whether we feel like participating at all. The hormonal changes during your menstrual cycle can affect how motivated you feel, how strong you are, how much stamina you have, and how quickly you recover – sometimes for the better, and sometimes not.[19] However, while your motivation and desire to move your body may be low during certain times of the cycle, there's good evidence that exercise can actually help relieve symptoms of painful periods and PMS.[20] [21] [22] [23] [24] Given the wide-ranging benefits of exercise, from stronger bones to healthier brains, it's essential to find ways to support girls and women in staying active throughout their menstrual cycle, even if that means adjusting the intensity of exercise, how much we do, the type of exercise we choose – or even what we wear.

PHYSICAL ACTIVITY VS EXERCISE

'Physical activity' and 'exercise' are often used interchangeably, but they aren't exactly the same. While exercise is a form of physical activity, it is not the only form.

Physical activity includes all kinds of movements that use energy, like walking the dog, cycling to work, gardening, or playing with kids. Exercise is a specific type of physical activity that's planned and repetitive, like going to a yoga class, running or lifting weights, with the goal of improving or maintaining fitness.

It's important to recognize this difference, because focusing only on structured exercise can make staying active seem less achievable for everyone. The key message is that *all* **movement** counts. Whether it's a casual walk or a gym session, any activity is better than none. This inclusive approach makes it easier for people of all abilities to stay active and healthy.

How the menstrual cycle impacts your workouts

Before we get into this next section, I want you to ask yourself: 'Is there a point in your cycle at which you find you perform best?'

When 195 Australian female athletes taking part in the 2020 Olympic and Paralympic Games were asked a similar question, 42 per cent said 'just after [the] period' as an ideal training window.[25] A smaller percentage preferred different times of the month and 23 per cent felt unsure when they would prefer. I was so surprised about that last statistic, but I think this highlights a really important point: when it comes to how you feel during sport and exercise throughout your menstrual cycle, you might not notice any changes at all, or the changes you do notice might not align with what the research says. The more I learn about the menstrual cycle and how it impacts women's bodies, the more I begin to understand how every cycle is different and how unique each of our experiences can be.

Let's take a look at what the research says about how your body handles exercise and recovery during different phases of your menstrual cycle, and how we can use this knowledge to enhance our training goals and overall health.

Menstruation

The period . . .

Research suggests there might be a small drop in strength and endurance (or your energy to keep going!) when your period first starts, compared to other times in your menstrual cycle.[26] However, the difference is likely small and some studies have found no changes at all. One interesting study found that while female athletes felt worse during their period, and believed that this negatively impacted their performance, their reaction times were actually faster and they made fewer errors during this time.[27] I caution against interpreting this as 'it's all in her head' and rather: **how we feel doesn't always reflect how we perform**. That said, even if actual performance measures don't change much, a lot of women feel like they're not at their best during their period and right before it starts. So give yourself a break if the only marathons you want to think about right now are on Netflix.[28]

Motivation to work out is also typically lower during this time (I know you don't need me to tell you that), and sometimes women feel that exercise requires more effort than usual.[29] You might feel like you're pushing yourself more, breathing heavier, and your legs feel heavier, even though you're running at your usual pace or lifting weights you normally lift. Plus, delayed onset muscle soreness (DOMS) can be more intense, so stiff and sore muscles, combined with menstrual symptoms like pain, bloating and bleeding, can really affect how you feel and your desire to exercise.[30]

All of that said, regular movement can actually reduce the risk of painful periods by acting as a natural pain reliever and lowering levels of pain-causing chemicals called prostaglandins.[31] A 2019 review found that doing 45–60 minutes of exercise (at any intensity) at least 3 times a week really helped reduce menstrual cramps, cut down the need for painkillers, and lowered the chances of missing school or work.[32] Unfortunately it's unlikely to work if you only do it now and then, as most studies show it takes 8–12 weeks of regular exercise to start seeing benefits. It's also unclear if those benefits last if you stop exercising regularly.[33] [34]

Practicing yoga (*asanas/pranayama/yoga nidra*) is one form of movement that seems to be particularly helpful if you struggle with painful periods.[35] Yoga helps by boosting blood flow to the pelvis, lowering stress hormones, and relaxing your pelvic muscles through deep breathing and long exhalations.[36] Even if you're no yogi, I've pulled some beginner-friendly yoga poses from the studies that you can come back to if you're dealing with period cramps.

SOME YOGA POSES TO TRY FOR PERIOD PAIN RELIEF:

CAT POSE (MARJARIASANA)

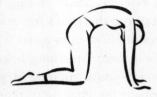

BOUND ANGLE POSE (BADDHA KONASANA)

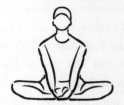

FISH POSE (MATSYASANA)

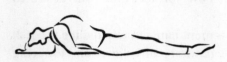

LOTUS POSE (PADMASANA)

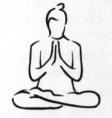

COBRA POSE (BHUJANGASANA)

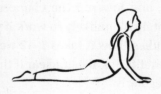

BOAT POSE (NAVASANA)

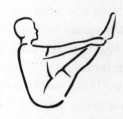

BRIDGE POSE (SETU BANDHASANA)

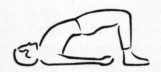

HARE POSE (SHASHANKASANA)

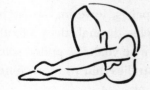

Late follicular phase and ovulation

the days following the period . . .

Oestrogen can help build muscle, increasing both strength and size, and it plays a key role in muscle repair and recovery, including reducing the soreness you often feel the day after a workout, known as DOMS.[37][38] Progesterone is believed to counteract some of the benefits of oestrogen, so when oestrogen is high and progesterone is low during the late follicular phase (after your period and before ovulation), it might give a boost to your strength and energy in your workouts.[39] Some studies suggest that doing more resistance training during your follicular phase (the first half of your cycle) is better for building strength and muscle than training during your luteal phase (the second half) or sticking to a regular routine.[40][41][42][43][44] Around ovulation, testosterone levels peak slightly, which might also help improve strength and performance. This is because testosterone helps build muscle and can also increase motivation and the drive to compete.[45][46][47]

That said, while some studies suggest you might be stronger during this time (and you might feel it!), a recent large review, which looks at a lot of past research, found that there's no solid evidence showing the menstrual cycle phase affects strength, muscle size or strength gains.[48] Many people were interested in my opinion on this study, and to be honest, I wasn't surprised by its findings – this is not the first paper to come to this conclusion, and I'm sure not the last, as the research in this space is sparse, typically poorly designed and often conflicting.* I firmly believe that while research can guide us, the most important piece of evidence comes from collecting data from *your* own menstrual cycle and understanding how it affects how *you* feel and perform in the activities you

---

* Beginning to notice a theme, here? Yep, me too.

enjoy – whether it's going to the gym, taking a walk, swimming, or playing team sports.

When reading research on the menstrual cycle, keep in mind that a lot of studies assume everyone has the same 'textbook' cycle, like ovulating on day 14, without actually checking hormone levels.[49][50] This can make the research less reliable and not always true of real-life people like you and I.

This is why I believe cookie-cutter workout programmes based on the menstrual cycle aren't practical or evidence-based. Since everyone's cycle is different, not all will experience noticeable changes in how they respond to or recover from exercise. While these menstrual-cycle-based programmes are becoming popular, especially with fitness influencers and apps, they're too generic and could potentially lead to not getting enough exercise, particularly in strength training due to an emphasis on rest, recovery and low-intensity movement. Instead, use the information here, along with your own cycle data and symptoms, to guide your workouts. This might mean adjusting weights, switching out uncomfortable exercises, or taking it easy when you're not feeling your best.

HOW MUCH PHYSICAL ACTIVITY DO WE NEED TO DO TO GAIN HEALTH BENEFITS?

All adults (both men and women, and whether you menstruate or not) are advised to do:

* At least 150 minutes of moderate-intensity aerobic activity (e.g., brisk walking, dancing) a week

* OR

* At least 75 minutes of vigorous-intensity aerobic activity (e.g., running, swimming laps, sports) a week

* PLUS

* **Muscle-strengthening activities** on 2 or more days a week (e.g., lifting weights, gymnastics, Pilates)

Additionally, I would also add that it is especially important for women to include:

* **Pelvic Floor Training**: Every day, at least once a day, and up to 2–3 times a day if you have pelvic floor dysfunction symptoms such as incontinence.

* **Weight-bearing activities**: Essentially, any activity where you are standing on one or both feet (jogging, hiking, jumping, dancing and most types of sports), as these appear to be the most effective at strengthening bones and maintaining bone health.

I know it can be tricky to find the time to fit movement in when juggling work, commuting and family commitments, but remember these are just guidelines, not the rule, and something is better than nothing. You might find it's easier to pair it up with things you already do. For example, perhaps squeeze in your pelvic floor training while the kettle boils or try walking some of your commute to work or the school pickup to get some steps in.

Luteal phase

After ovulation until the next period . . .

In the second half of the menstrual cycle, oestrogen levels (which previously dropped off at ovulation) rise again. However, progesterone also rises and peaks mid-cycle, which may hamper some of oestrogen's strength and stamina benefits by increasing body temperature and affecting how your body responds to stress and physical activity.[51] [52]

These negative effects seem to show up more when you're working out in hot conditions or pushing yourself to the max (like doing sprints).[53] [54] [55] For example, during treadmill tests at different effort levels, it was found that running economy – how efficiently your body uses energy while running – was lower in the mid-luteal phase compared to the follicular phase. This means you might feel like you're working harder to maintain the same pace during the mid-luteal phase.[56] Similarly, for a group of female football players, their performance on a beep test was noticeably lower during the luteal phase compared to the follicular phase.[57] Conversely, another study found that more runners had their best marathon times during the luteal phase than in the follicular phase. They didn't consider factors like weather, terrain or the course, however, all of which has a big impact on how well we run.[58] I think this just goes to show that the menstrual cycle isn't the only thing affecting our performance. Things like environment, heat, nutrition, recovery and how hard you work out also play a big role.

If you wear a smartwatch that measures heart rate variability (HRV) and resting heart rate (RHR), you might have noticed that they change across the menstrual cycle too. HVR is a measure of the time between your heartbeats, and in simple terms, it shows how well your body is handling stress and how quickly it can recover. A higher HRV usually means your body is more relaxed and recovering well, while a lower HRV can indicate stress, or that your body needs more rest. The opposite is true of RHR, where a lower score is generally a good sign of your fitness level, overall health and recovery from exercise. If it's higher than normal, it might be a sign that your body is still stressed or needs more time to recover from previous workouts or a period of stress.

From one period ending to the next, we typically see HRV slowly go down and RHR slowly go up, which indicates recovery might be reduced.[59] [60] Once the next period starts, these numbers often recover or start to improve. I personally have noticed this with my own wearable data, and until I understood why, I used to think I was about to come down with the flu almost every month! Now that I understand why these changes happen, however, I no longer panic or worry that I'm suddenly 'unhealthy', and instead, it allows me to be more compassionate towards myself and signals that now might be a good time to double down on recovery, sleep and good nutrition to support my body.

Another reason you might want to reduce the intensity of your workouts or opt for more gentle forms of movement like swimming or walking during the end of the luteal phase is that this is when premenstrual symptoms like irritability, anxiety, bloating and breast tenderness often start to kick in. Plus, sleep can be disrupted during this time, affecting your focus and energy during exercise. However, light to moderate exercise might actually help with these symptoms, so if you're feeling up to it, staying active can be good for both your body and mind.[61] [62] It's important to say that some women feel fine during this time and, if that's you, then crack on as normal.

Throughout your menstrual cycle, you might notice feeling stronger, more motivated, or more energetic at different times. The research on this is limited and often mixed – some studies show changes in how you exercise and recover, while others don't see any difference. But just because the evidence isn't clear doesn't mean your experiences aren't real. In the end, you know your body better than anyone, so pay attention to how you feel and use any advice as a guide, not a hard rule.

Impact of the pill on strength, exercise and recovery

Compared to a natural menstrual cycle, the combined oral contraceptive pill (COCPs) might slightly impact exercise performance, but the difference is pretty minor.[63] And whether you're on a pill-taking day or a pill-free day doesn't seem to make much of a difference either.[64] The impact of hormonal contraceptives (HCs) on strength training results is a bit of a mixed bag: some studies show positive effects, others show negative effects, and some find no difference at all compared to women who menstruate naturally.

Since the combined pill works by altering the body's natural production of oestrogen and progesterone, you might think it would reduce the strength-promoting benefits of natural oestrogen. But the research doesn't really back that up, and overall, it seems like the pill doesn't have a significant effect on muscle growth, power or strength gains from strength training.[65]

As for recovery, using the combined pill might slightly slow down recovery compared to naturally menstruating women, with some trends showing lower muscle strength, higher levels of creatine kinase (a marker of muscle damage) and increased muscle soreness.[66] But most of the research has focused on the combined pill, so we need more studies on other types of hormonal contraceptives to fully understand their impact. We also don't know much about how the pill and other forms of hormonal contraception impact other forms of movement outside of strength and endurance training.

In a nutshell, some women might find the pill affects their performance, strength or recovery, while others don't notice a difference. It's super individual, so the best way to know is to track how you feel and see what works for you.

How your workouts influence the menstrual cycle

We looked at some of the ways our menstrual cycle can impact our performance, recovery and participation in sport and exercise – but it's a two-way relationship, and how often, or how hard, we exercise, and how we fuel our sessions, can also have a knock-on effect on our menstrual cycle and our overall health.

While regular exercise can help reduce the risk of painful periods and alleviate PMS symptoms like pain, fatigue, mood swings and bloating, it's important we are adequately fuelling our training sessions with enough calories.[67] As we discussed in the previous chapter, overexercising and/or not consuming enough calories can lead to period loss. Consequently, many women who are dedicated gym-goers, runners or triathletes often end up in my DMs asking why their periods have become irregular or have stopped altogether. If this has happened to you, or you've just embarked on a new fitness journey and want to avoid this, keep reading. This is more common than you might think and a study of regular exercising women found that half had menstrual disturbances and over a third had no period at all.[68]

The mismatch between calorie intake and energy expenditure, known as low energy availability (LEA), can manifest as a condition known as relative energy deficiency in sport, or RED-S for short. Period loss or irregular cycles is often the first (or the most obvious) symptom, but it is only alerting us to a larger, system-wide problem in the body.

Relative Energy Deficiency in Sport (RED-S)

RED-S is a condition that can affect almost every part of your body, including your heart, bones, hormones, metabolism and immune system.[69] This doesn't just mean your performance in sports or exercise might suffer – it also means your body isn't functioning as well as it should, leading to a higher risk of fractures, injuries, infections, and feeling more irritable or down.[70] [71] The term RED-S has replaced the old 'female athlete triad' (which focused on low energy, period loss and low bone density) because it affects both men and women and goes far beyond just menstrual and bone health.

Reduced Immunity (weakened ability to fight off illnesses)
Impaired Reproductive Function (irregular or absent periods)

Impaired Bone Health (weakened bones and higher risk of fractures)

Impaired Gastrointestinal Function (gut issues like bloating or discomfort)

Impaired Energy Metabolism (resting metabolic rate is reduced in order to conserve energy)

Impaired Haematological Function (issues with blood health, like low iron or anaemia)

Urinary Incontinence (difficulty controlling bladder)

Impaired Glucose & Lipid Metabolism (problems blood sugar regulation and cholesterol levels)

Mental Health Issues (increased risk of anxiety and depression)

Impaired Neurocognitive Function (trouble concentrating or thinking clearly)

Sleep Disturbances (difficulty sleeping or poor-quality sleep)

Impaired Cardiovascular Function (heart and circulation problems)

Reduced Skeletal Muscle Function (reduced strength)

Impaired Growth & Development (slowed growth or delayed physical development, especially in younger individuals)

While RED-S is often associated with athletes, it can actually happen to anyone, even if you're just working out casually. It's not always intentional, either – we might not realize how much energy we're burning during workouts, which can create a deficit without us even noticing. If you're worried that's happening or has happened to you, do reach out to a medical doctor or registered dietitian working in this field for support. And remember, a nourished body is a strong and resilient body.

Case Study: Olivia

Olivia, a 37-year-old new mum to a two-year-old, reached out after losing her period and having been given a suspected diagnosis of relative energy deficiency in sport (RED-S). This occurred a few months postpartum, when she started running and reducing her calorie intake to lose some weight that she had gained during pregnancy. Her weight went from 89kg (14 stone) to 66kg (10 stone 3lbs), causing her periods, which were initially on a regular 28-day cycle after giving birth, to become irregular. Her GP arranged blood tests, which showed that essentially all of her reproductive hormone levels were low. Her goal was to improve the regularity of her cycles with plans to conceive again.

To help Olivia get her cycle back on track, we focused on a few key areas:

✳ *Increasing calories and ensuring regular meal timings, with three meals and three snacks per day.*

✳ *Embracing and not fearing carbs as a source of energy, regardless of activity levels.*

✳ *Adding more nutrient-rich foods like avocados, nuts, fatty fish, full-fat dairy and olive oil to her diet, to increase calories and nutrients.*

✳ *Reducing running from 6 runs per week to 2 times per week and cutting out high-intensity workouts.*

We also focused on stress management techniques to help regulate her cycle and overall wellbeing.

Since making these changes, Olivia has seen some great progress.

Her cycles are now 29 days in length, arriving every month, and she has confirmation of ovulation using ovulation sticks.

This case study shows RED-S and period loss can happen to anyone, regardless of whether you're a professional athlete or a mum just trying to get in shape.

TO PREVENT RUNNING LOW:

* **Match your energy intake to your energy output:** If you increase how much exercise you're doing (if you've just signed up to a half marathon, for example), make sure you adjust your nutrition intake accordingly.

* **Aim to have regular balanced meals:** Include protein, carbohydrates and fats, and avoid skipping meals, fasted training or prolonged periods of time without eating.

* **Don't forget your micronutrients:** Ensure you have adequate intake of key micronutrients, such as vitamin D and calcium for bone health and iron for oxygen transport and energy production.[72] Women are at greater risk of iron deficiency anaemia due to iron losses during menstruation, but active women, especially runners, have a greater risk due to losses through sweat, hemolysis (destruction of red blood cells due to the repetitive impact of foot strikes), gut losses and inflammation.[73]

* **Prioritize and optimize nutrition around your training sessions:** See point below. *Note: appetite is not always indicative of your food and fuelling needs.*

* **Rest days require fuel too!** Energy is needed not just for performance but also for recovery and overall health. Reducing your intake, especially of important nutrients like carbohydrates, on rest days can leave you depleted for your next training session, negatively affecting your performance.
* **Seek professional guidance:** Consult a dietitian or registered nutritionist if you think you are experiencing LEA or RED-S.

Check out page X for signs and symptoms of low energy availability (LEA) to learn more.

Fuelling your cycle

To avoid running into a low energy state and ensure you're eating enough to fuel your workouts, pay attention to how you feel during and after your workouts, as well as in your daily life. If you're feeling exhausted, struggling through your training and taking longer to recover, it might mean you're not getting enough energy – also keep an eye out for LEA red flags (page x). On the other hand, if you feel energized throughout the day, recover well and see progress in your training, you're likely fuelling your body properly.

Before your workouts

Have a meal (3–4 hours before) or a snack (~2 hours before) to give your body time to digest and avoid gut issues like bloating or nausea. Focus on carbohydrates, with some protein and minimal fat. Carbs are the main energy source for exercise, and too much fat can slow digestion and cause gut symptoms during your workout.

Some ideas might be:

* Overnight oats made with oats, chia seeds, milk, yoghurt and berries

* Chicken or tofu wrap with veggies and hummus
* Bagel with smoked salmon or scrambled eggs
* Crumpets or toast with honey or jam
* Flapjack or a cereal bar
* A banana

During your workouts

If you exercise for less than 60 minutes, water is usually sufficient. For workouts longer than 60–90 minutes, start fuelling with 30–60g of carbs per hour after 45–60 minutes to sustain blood glucose levels and conserve glycogen stores; for endurance activities over 2.5 hours, increase intake to up to 90g of mixed carbohydrates per hour.

Examples of food with (roughly) 30g of carbohydrates:

* 1 large banana
* 500ml sports drink
* 1–1.5 gels (most gels contain 20–25g carbs)
* ~ 6 jelly babies
* 1 cereal or oat-based energy bar
* 2 large medjool dates

After your workouts

When it comes to recovery nutrition, remember the 4 'R's:

* Refuel with carbohydrates
* Repair with protein
* Rehydrate with fluids
* Renourish with antioxidant-rich foods (e.g., colourful fruit and veggies)

Note: Fats, while not part of the 4 'R's, are still super important in the diet for overall health, but especially so for hormone production and the prevention of LEA.

Some meal ideas might be:

* A smoothie with oats, berries, peanut butter, protein powder or yoghurt
* A black bean burrito
* Chicken stir fry with veggies and rice
* A baked sweet potato with tuna and sweetcorn
* Flavoured milk and a cereal bar

Summary

* Hormonal fluctuations might impact motivation, strength, endurance and recovery.
  * Menstruation: Potential dip in performance and motivation, and increase in DOMS and perceived effort.
  * Late follicular phase: Strength and muscle-building potential may be enhanced.
  Luteal phase: Recovery may drop off and performance may be impaired especially when exercising in hot conditions and when working close to maximal intensities.

* Regular physical activity can help alleviate period pain and PMS.
* The combined oral contraceptive pill (COCP) might slightly reduce exercise performance and recovery, but the effect is minimal.
* Overexercising and under-fuelling can lead to period loss and RED-S (relative energy deficiency in sport), affecting overall health and performance.

Sleep

As we go about our daily lives, it's easy to overlook the importance of one of the most fundamental aspects of our health: sleep. Despite its central role in our overall wellbeing, many of us treat rest as an afterthought, sacrificing precious hours of shut-eye in the name of productivity, success and 'the hustle'. But the truth is, our bodies (yes, that includes our hormones) need sleep just as much as they need proper nutrition, regular exercise and relaxation. Without it, we're more vulnerable to everything from mental health issues to chronic illnesses – not to mention period problems.

I'm not going to lie, in the past, I didn't fully appreciate the importance of sleep. I used to think of it as a passive activity that simply recharges our bodies after a long day. As a medical student and NHS doctor, sleep was often sidelined by early morning ward rounds and late-night studying – or partying, depending on the day. I convinced myself that I was one of the few people who could function well on just a few hours of sleep. It's now a running joke that when I first met my partner, I smugly told him that I only needed 5–6 hours of sleep. However, when I'm left to sleep undisturbed, I can easily sleep for a good 8–9 hours, and aim to do so most nights. If I knew then what I know now – if I had, in fact, slept more – I would have consolidated more of what I had learned in lectures and performed better at university and work, and had more energy for everyday life. That said, I also understand that not everyone has the luxury of choosing how much sleep they get. For those with young children, shift-workers , or those who have to travel for work , getting enough sleep – or good-quality sleep – is often easier said than done. It's a reminder that sleep isn't just a personal choice but something we need to prioritize as best we can within the realities of our lives.

Despite what I may have believed in the past, sleep is far from a passive process: it is essential to every function in the body, affecting our physical and mental performance, immune system, metabolism and, of course, our menstrual cycle. The duration, timing and quality of sleep can all influence the menstrual cycle. For example, women who sleep less than 6 hours per night are more likely to report irregular menstrual cycles.[1] [2] And the relationship goes both ways: not only can sleep impact the menstrual cycle, but the menstrual cycle can influence how we sleep. In our research survey, 70 per cent of women reported decreased sleep quality related to their menstrual cycle and 66 per cent reported that it disrupted their daily activities to some degree. This is often worse at certain times of the cycle, in particular just before and during menstruation – and those who experience painful periods (dysmenorrhoea) and PMS are more likely to be affected.[3]

Understanding how your sleep may be disturbed during certain phases of the menstrual cycle is an important first step to better rest – and, as we've just learned, a healthy amount of sleep supports a healthy cycle. Before learning about how sleep impacts the menstrual cycle (and vice versa), however, it's important we get to grips with the basics of sleep.

The basics of sleep

Sleep can be divided into two types – rapid eye movement (REM) and non-rapid eye movement (non-REM).

The main difference between REM and non-REM sleep is the level of brain activity, eye movement and muscle control.

REM sleep is characterized by rapid eye movement, increased brain activity and vivid dreams. REM sleep plays a role in memory consolidation, emotional processing, brain development and dreaming.

Non-REM sleep is characterized by slowed brain activity, breathing and heart rate, and reduced eye movement. Non-REM sleep can be further divided into four stages, each stage representing a deeper level of sleep. Non-REM sleep stages are vital for physical and mental restoration.

Your body cycles through these stages four to five times each night. Although non-REM sleep usually makes up the majority of our total sleep time, the ratio of REM to non-REM sleep varies throughout the night. For example, we tend to experience most of our deep non-REM sleep earlier in the night (stages 3 and 4), while REM sleep dominates the latter part of the night. Since you get most of your REM sleep in the second half of the night, short sleepers tend to get less of it. Often people think of deep sleep as the best sleep or an indicator of a good night's sleep, but each phase is integral to your overall wellbeing, whether you're experiencing deep non-REM sleep or vivid dream-filled REM sleep.

A good night's sleep might be summarized by the following statements:[4]

* You fall asleep easily (in 30 minutes or less)
* You do not wake up during the night (or no more than once)

* If you do wake up, you fall back asleep in under 20 minutes

* You can sleep a full 7–9 hours per night

* You wake up in the morning feeling refreshed

Diagram to follow

Adapted from: Charlotte Ruhl. 5 Stages of Sleep. *Simply Psychology* (2023)[5]

Sleep and hormones

Do women need more sleep than men? Perhaps. Science suggests women tend to sleep slightly longer than men (just over 11 minutes) but they also tend to have worse-quality sleep overall, including difficulty falling asleep, waking up frequently in the night and having longer wakeful episodes.[6][7] Women are also at higher risk of insomnia, and this difference emerges around the time of puberty (hint: hormones are at play).[8] Periods of hormonal shifts that occur during the menstrual cycle, pregnancy and during the menopause transition can also contribute to poor sleep and are times when sleep disorders such as insomnia and restless legs syndrome can emerge.[9]

This is in part due to hormones, but the role of sex hormones, such as oestrogen and progesterone, in sleep is not yet fully understood – and a little confusing! Overall, oestrogen appears to have a positive effect on sleep and is associated with better sleep efficiency and less awakenings during the night.[10][11] It also helps to regulate body temperature at night, keeping us cool, which is important for a restful night's sleep. This is particularly relevant during perimenopause and menopause, when hot flashes – caused by fluctuating and lower levels of oestrogen – can wreak havoc on sleep.[12] [13]

Progesterone is thought to support sleep in other ways, but its role appears to be more variable. For example, a sharp decrease in progesterone in the late luteal phase is associated with sleep disruption.[14] On the other hand, other studies have found that higher levels of progesterone actually lead to worse sleep and more time awake during the night.[15] [16] So, while higher oestrogen levels generally enhance sleep quality, the effects of progesterone are more inconsistent. Elevated progesterone levels (as seen in the mid-luteal phase) and lower levels (during the late luteal phase or menstruation) have both been associated with poorer sleep quality.

Of course, hormones are not the only thing at play here, and other factors like co-existing health conditions and social norms also influence sleep. For example, women are more likely to experience overactive bladder (OAB), meaning they typically wake up more times in the night to use the toilet[17] [18] and are more likely to suffer with depression and anxiety, as well as chronic pain, all of which impact sleep. Another important factor to consider is how gendered social roles and cultural norms are also tied up in this. Women disproportionately act as informal caregivers for children, older adults and relatives, which means less time for sleep and more sleep interruptions.[19]

So do women need *more* sleep in order to counteract all of these sleep disruptors? I think it depends on you and your individual situation. It's clear that women typically have more fragmented sleep throughout the night, but this is due to various reasons – not just our biology – so it's important to look at the bigger picture and consider other factors at play. However, it's not all in your head if you find yourself having cyclical sleep problems at certain times in your cycle. Personally, I like to track my sleep using a wearable device, and with that I've been able to find clear patterns in my sleep and recovery, related to the menstrual cycle. So I know when to expect some sleep disruption and I am able to proactively incorporate helpful sleep hygiene practices to offset it as much as possible (see page xx).

Sleep and the menstrual cycle

'My sleep is massively affected leading up to and during my period. I get insomnia and really struggle to sleep. I feel unsettled and anxious and get terrible night sweats, which means disturbed sleep. It's difficult, as the lack of sleep makes me irritable and then I crave more sugar. A vicious cycle! Sleep is so important to me as I am a very active person and bad sleep affects my performance with my running and strength training.' – Maya, 37

It probably comes as no surprise that sleep disturbance is common in the days leading up to and during menstruation.[20] [21] [22] This is thought to be due to body temperature changes, premenstrual cramps and other symptoms related to hormone fluctuations that can reduce the quality of your sleep. However, some women may also experience sleep disturbances mid-cycle, just after ovulation when the body temperature rises by approximately 0.5-1 degree.[23] It is worth noting that some women report no issues sleeping at any point in their menstrual cycle – and if that's you, that's awesome.

Not only does the menstrual cycle influence how much sleep we get, but it may also influence the type of sleep. During the luteal phase, when progesterone is high, there is reduced REM sleep, which is thought to be related to a higher body temperature during this time.[24] Matthew Walker, author of *Why We Sleep*, calls REM sleep 'emotional first aid', which may explain, in part, why we can feel a bit more irritable during this time.[25] In studies examining brain waves during sleep, it has been shown that, in the luteal phase, there are increased sleep spindles – which are essentially a specific pattern of brain waves that occur during sleep.[26] The interesting thing is that sleep spindles are thought to *support* sleep quality, and so their increased activity in the luteal phase may be a mechanism to maintain sleep quality as best as possible while we experience these disruptive hormonal fluctuations late in the cycle.[27]

While some of this is biologically driven by our hormones, we can't forget those pesky cramps keeping us up too. And while we don't really need a science journal to tell us this, evidence shows that when period pain is severe, it negatively impacts sleep, including the quality of sleep, daytime sleepiness and lower sleep efficiency (the ratio between the time you are actually asleep and the total time in bed).[28] This is also true of PMS and PMDD, but in this case, poor sleep quality may also be influenced by mood-related symptoms like anxiety and depression.[29] That said, women with PMDD seem to have a decreased response to melatonin (the hormone that helps induce sleep) in their luteal phase compared to the follicular phase, and therefore supplementing with melatonin may be helpful for women with PMDD.[30] [31] Unfortunately, these supplements are not authorized for sale in the UK and it's a prescription-only medicine.

Other factors, like worrying about leaking at night, can keep us up too. One study of female college students found that they are more likely to have less deep sleep during their period when they're concerned about sanitary products.[32] This highlights how important it is to have comfortable and reliable period products at night, such as high-absorbency period pants, menstrual cups and sanitary towels (see page x).

Just like the menstrual cycle can mess with your sleep, sleep (or lack thereof) can mess with your cycle. Short sleep duration and poor sleep quality are associated with irregular cycles, heavier bleeding and increased PMS symptoms.[33] [34] One study found that women who get less than 6 hours of sleep on average per night were 44 per cent more likely to have an irregular period and 70 per cent more likely to have heavy periods than women who got 7–9 hours of sleep.[35] I realize the opportunity for sleep is not the same for everyone, and as someone who used to do *many* night shifts as a junior doctor, I found stats like this pretty hard to swallow. It's an unfortunate truth, however, that shift work is not great for our overall health – including our menstrual cycle.[36] [37] [38]

Shift work and the menstrual cycle

Shift work is thought to disrupt the menstrual cycle by impacting the sex hormones that control it, and also by disrupting the body's circadian rhythm (also known as the 'internal body clock'), which in turn alters how our biological processes work, including our hormones.[39] [40] [41] On top of this, generally, people working at night are exposed to noise, light and stress – not to mention the lack of sleep – which can also interfere with normal physiology and lead to menstrual cycle disturbances.[42] If you are a night-shift worker, I don't want you to panic reading this, and it's important to understand that the risk is not the same for everyone. Shift work is also associated with poor lifestyle factors, such as smoking and physical inactivity, which we can control and modify to the best of our ability.

Tips for shift-workers:

* **Aim to get 7 hours of sleep in 24 hours:** When working nights, your days should be spent mostly sleeping – speak to friends, family and neighbours and tell them when you're working nights so they don't disrupt your schedule. While getting the full 7–9 hours of recommended sleep per night can be tricky, this doesn't have to be in one block and can be broken into shorter sleep periods.
* **Develop a bedtime routine:** Choose activities that promote relaxation before bed, such as mediation, reading and

mindfulness activities. Usual sleep hygiene tips apply, so aim to keep your bedroom cool, dark and quiet (eye masks, blackout blinds and ear plugs are your best friends).

* **Consider caffeine intake:** Having caffeine before work or at the start of your shift will help you feel alert, but try to avoid it for the second half of your shift so that it doesn't impact your sleep when you get home.

* **Meal timing:** Where possible, opt for smaller, protein-rich meals or snacks during night shifts (e.g., hard-boiled eggs, yoghurt, protein shake) and have your main meals before and after your shifts. Sip on water throughout the shift, as dehydration can lead to fatigue and reduce mental alertness.

* **Selective light exposure:** Exposure to bright light before bed can impact your sleep (which is pretty hard to avoid if your job involves looking at a screen all night!). Expose yourself to natural light before work and wear sunglasses on the way home after a night shift.

* **Remain active:** Regular exercise can help improve sleep quality and is also beneficial for offsetting other risks associated with shift work. Research now shows that exercise before bed, unless it's high intensity and less than an hour before, doesn't disrupt sleep for most people.[43]

Advice for parents of young children

I'm always conscious of parents with young children when discussing sleep hygiene tips, as sometimes it can create more anxiety when you've already got a lot on your plate. How much sleep you get in the early months and years depends a fair bit on what's happening with your baby, and the support you have around you. If you can, share baby care with your partner, so you both feel as rested as possible. A family member or friend might be able to help too. Taking turns or shifts for night-time duties, or 6am starts with toddlers, can make a difference. This might be harder for breastfeeding mothers and, in this case, try to rest when your baby is resting. While the amount of sleep you get may vary, try to optimize the quality of the hours you do get by finding ways to switch off before bed, like having a warm shower or reading a book, and avoiding stimulants like tea or coffee in the afternoon.

Sleep and hormonal contraception

At this point you might be thinking, what does this mean for me if I'm taking the pill? Well, we can't say for sure, as there are only a handful of studies exploring this, and they've generally been done on only small groups of women.

A 2020 study surveyed over 2,000 women and found that hormonal contraceptive users had more insomnia symptoms and increased levels of daytime sleepiness compared to non-users.[44] Interestingly, people using progestogen-only methods reported sleeping less in total compared with those on a combined type.[45] However, earlier studies found that hormonal contraceptive users had fewer awakenings during the night and better sleep efficiency.[46] [47] So, we can't say for sure!

Then, looking at the type of sleep, also known as sleep architecture, women taking oral contraceptives have also been found to have less deep, slow-wave sleep and more stage 2 light sleep compared to those not using them.[48] [49] [50] However, it's not known if the changes affect how these women feel when they're awake, and they may not notice it at all.

All of that said, some women might find they sleep better on the pill or other forms of hormonal contraception, especially if they suffer from disruptive symptoms like painful or heavy periods. The bottom line is, hormonal contraception may impact sleep, but if it does, it's likely small.

How to sleep better across your menstrual cycle

If, like me, you notice that your sleep is pretty rubbish in the nights leading up to or during your period (or at any point during the cycle), here are some tips to give you the best chance at a good night's sleep:

1. **Monitor your menstrual cycle:** Be aware of how your menstrual cycle affects your individual sleep patterns by tracking them – because everyone is different. Understanding these patterns can allow you to be proactive at doubling down on your positive sleep habits during times of sleep disruption.
2. **Address pain and discomfort:** Take steps to alleviate any discomfort that may interfere with sleep, such as painful cramps. This might include pain killers, using hot-water bottles or heat pads, having a warm bath or finding comfortable sleeping positions. Anecdotally, sleeping in the foetal position can often help, as it encourages the tummy muscles to relax, which may reduce the intensity of menstrual cramps.
3. **Adjust your sleep environment:** In the days leading up to your period, you may be more sensitive to temperature changes and body temperature fluctuations. Ensure your bedroom is cool and comfortable, and consider using breathable bedding and loose, cotton or bamboo pyjamas.
4. **Consider menstrual products:** Choose comfortable and reliable menstrual products, whether it's using overnight pads, menstrual cups or period underwear, to help you feel more relaxed and confident during sleep.
5. Usual sleep hygiene tips apply!

   - Try to stick to a consistent, regular sleep routine, going to bed and waking up at the same time every day. This helps regulate your body's internal clock, making it easier to fall asleep and wake up feeling refreshed.

- Reduce exposure to screens (phones, computers, TVs) before bed, as the blue light can disrupt your sleep–wake cycle. Dim overhead lights and use low-lighting lamps and candles instead.
- Create a sleep-friendly environment by keeping your bedroom cool, dark and quiet.
- Wind down before bed with calming activities like reading, meditation or taking a warm bath. This signals to your body that it's time to unwind and prepare for sleep.
- Aim to have your last meal 2–3 hours before bed, avoiding large portions, spicy or fatty foods late in the evening.
- Cut out caffeine after midday. The half-life (time taken to eliminate half of the caffeine in your system) varies from person to person, but can be anywhere from 2 to 10 hours.[51]

LEAKING AT NIGHT

Leaking at night during your period is not a fun experience, but it is pretty common for a few reasons:

* Firstly, you're asleep for a long time, likely longer than you would normally go before checking or changing your pad or tampon. This means it's even more important to choose a menstrual product that has high absorbency and change it right before you go to bed.

* Being horizontal for so long means gravity will make your menstrual fluid fall to one side of your underwear or another. We can't defy gravity, but adding a mattress protector can be helpful to prevent stains (and your peace of mind).

* If you're someone who tends to move about a lot when you sleep, this can cause your underwear/pad to bunch up, leading to leaks. Look for pads with wings or period pants that have good coverage.

Remember, if it does happen, there's no shame – periods are a natural part of life!

Note: If you find yourself leaking regularly at night, it could be a sign of heavy periods. See page x for more.

Summary

* Women tend to sleep slightly longer than men, though they typically have worse-quality sleep overall, including difficulty falling asleep, waking up frequently in the night and having longer wakeful episodes.

* The hormones oestrogen and progesterone play a role in the quality and architecture of our sleep – but they're not the only influencing factor.

* Sleep duration, timing and quality can influence the menstrual cycle.

* Sleep disturbance is more common at certain times of the cycle, in particular just before and during menstruation.

* Those who experience painful periods (dysmenorrhoea) and PMS/PMDD are more likely to experience problems with sleep.

* Hormonal contraception may impact sleep, but if it does, it's thought to be non-significant.

Mood

Picture this: You're 13 years old sitting in French class and the boy sitting behind you keeps flicking little paper balls into your hair. Pretty annoying, right? Well, I was that 13-year-old girl and I, quite rightly, snapped at the boy in question. But, for context, I rarely spoke up or stood up for myself in my early teenage years, so I guess this boy and his mates didn't expect it from me. Initially stunned by the fightback, the paper-flicking boy replied with a mocking, 'Oooooh, *someone* is on her period', which caused the whole class to burst into laughter. I've never felt so mortified, and I wish I could say that was the last time I was accused of being 'hormonal' after expressing emotion, but it certainly wasn't. It's as if, when you have a menstrual cycle, your anger, sadness or irritability are not valid emotional responses, and are always hormonally driven?

That said, it is true that our hormones can influence our mood and mental health, so it's not all in your head if you find your emotions are tightly connected to your cycle. However, if you take only one thing from this chapter, let it be this: Just because you are at a certain point in your cycle doesn't automatically mean that your emotional response was unjustified.

So, how about we stop blaming ourselves for being 'hormonal' and instead explore where these emotions are coming from and what they are trying to communicate?

How hormones influence mood

'I am very emotional from two days before my period through the first three days of bleeding. I also have quite irregular periods, so sometimes these mood swings and heightened emotions can last for a week or two depending on how irregular my period is than month. Around ovulation I have quite high energy and normally am in very good spirits. Sometimes, I feel extremely grateful and cry a lot of happy tears at this time!' – Angie, 24

Did you know women are twice as likely as men to develop depression during their lifetime – with a specific risk at puberty, the premenstrual part of the cycle, postpartum, and during the menopause transition?[1] In fact, women who are perimenopausal, with no prior history of depression, are 2 to 4 times more likely to develop depression than women in the premenopausal stage.[2] These periods of major hormonal shifts that many women go through across their lifespan create windows of vulnerability for mental health.

The relationship between hormones and mood is not fully understood. However, one way sex hormones are known to influence mood is by affecting specific chemical messengers in the brain, known as neurotransmitters. For example, there is a link between levels of oestrogen and levels of serotonin, which is often referred to as the 'happy hormone' due to its role in mood and wellbeing.[3] [4] Oestrogen has also been found to increase the levels of dopamine, which is known as the 'reward neurotransmitter' for its role in pleasure and motivation.[5] [6] This may explain why women typically report improved mood and motivation before ovulation, as oestrogen levels increase. Progesterone is believed to have calming and anti-anxiety effects, and so, as hormone levels plummet pre-menstruation, this may contribute to PMS symptoms of anxiety, irritability and mood disturbances. Other research suggests that women with PMDD (page xx) may have an increased sensitivity or altered response to progesterone and its metabolites, leading to negative mood symptoms.[7][8][9] This might be compared to how some people feel happy after having a drink, while others may feel angry or down.

It's important to note that most of this research is based on animals, which has provided valuable insights. However, I don't need to tell you that mouse models can't fully capture the complexities of human behaviour and emotions. For example, after puberty, girls are twice as likely to be affected by depression as boys, and this continues into adulthood.[10][11] While these changes coincide with a surge in sex hormones, there is no firm evidence that hormones directly cause 'puberty blues'. Consider your own experience of puberty for a moment: not only were you riding a mega wave of sex hormones, but you were likely also dealing with body changes, a new school, perhaps parental divorce or losing grandparents, all while under academic pressure and navigating life as a teenager with crushes, bullies and real-life 'Mean Girls'. While this is a tricky time for boys and girls, studies show that girls tend to feel more pressure about their appearance from friends compared to boys, and they're also more likely to worry about being excluded based on how they look.[12][13] On top of that, girls often tie their self-worth more closely to academic success than boys do.[14]

Similarly, during perimenopause, erratic changes in hormones during this time may impact how women feel, but this period of life also often comes with many other changes, such as children growing up and moving out, career pressure, divorce and ageing parents – not to mention poor sleep and hot flashes – all of which can influence our mood and increase the risk of depression.

So, although hormones drive these major stages in the female lifespan, the relationship is much more complex than simply saying, 'This hormone causes low mood or depression.'

Hormonal contraception and mood

One of the most commonly reported side effects of hormonal contraception is mood changes. In one study, over 50 per cent of women reported mood changes and/or sexual side effects (such as loss of libido) related to hormonal contraception.[15] In the same study, 83 per cent said their healthcare provider did not mention the possibility of these side effects when prescribing.[16] This type of study was based on a survey, however, which can provide us with valuable information but cannot prove cause and effect (i.e., it doesn't tell us for sure that hormonal contraception drives mood changes). That said, we can't deny the link, and one of the most common reasons given for stopping the use of pills is changes in mood, so let's take a closer look at the data.[17]

Several studies have explored the link between hormonal contraception and mood, and the results have been, well . . . inconsistent – probably due to variations in study designs, methodologies and measurements of mood and mental health outcomes.

In a study of over a million women in Denmark, it was found that hormonal contraception users were more likely to be diagnosed with depression and be prescribed medication for this for the first time than people who were not on hormonal contraception.[18] The link was stronger for teenagers. Naturally, this caused a lot of panic among people, but looking at the numbers, the absolute risk was actually very small – 1 extra person received antidepressants out of 200 people using hormonal methods for a year. This study was also based on registry data and was not a rigorously controlled study, and because of this, there are some other important factors that influence the risk of depression that were not accounted for in the analysis, which means we can't make a causal link, but we can say there is an association.

In a more tightly controlled study, 340 women aged 18–35 were split into two groups, where one received the pill and the other a placebo. After 3 months of the study, there was no increase in depressive symptoms, but there was a decrease in general wellbeing in the pill-taking group.[19]

Not all studies have found negative effects of mood or quality of life when using hormonal contraception, and some have even found improvements in mood and fewer symptoms of depression and anxiety.[20] [21]

So, the research suggests some women find hormonal contraception impacts their mood, some don't notice a difference, and some find that it improves mood. The risk seems to depend on the age (e.g., higher in teenagers), type of contraception (certain types of synthetic progesterones seem to carry a higher risk),[22] [23] [24] and history of depression and anxiety (which appear to increase the risk of psychological side effects associated with hormonal contraception).[25]

The fact is, historically, mood-related effects of the pill are woefully under-researched. Evidence is building, however, and healthcare providers should be counselling women on these potential risks and side effects. My advice? Work closely with your GP to find a suitable form of contraception, if that's what you require, and trial and monitor how your body (and mind) responds to it. Remember, not all women experience negative mood effects related to hormonal contraception – but if you do, you're not alone, and there are a variety of options and alternatives you can try (see page xx for a guide to hormonal and non-hormonal contraception options).

How stress impacts the menstrual cycle

Just like hormones can influence our mood and emotions, stress can influence our hormones, and indeed our menstrual cycles.

Stress is the body's reaction to a perceived threat or challenge, causing physical and mental changes to help cope with the situation. It's not always bad; sometimes, a small amount of stress can be a powerful motivator and help us perform at our best (which is why many people find they are most productive just before a deadline!). However, the positive effects of stress largely relate to acute stress, which is short-lived and overcome quickly, rather than chronic stress, which lasts for a long period of time or keeps coming back. This can feel never-ending and all-encompassing, impacting both our mental and physical health – and our menstrual cycles.

If the stress is short-lived, you may notice your period is a few days late. However, if the stress is chronic or severe, it can lead to irregular periods or no periods at all. Psychological stress has also been linked to more painful periods and worse PMS symptoms.

How chronic stress impacts the menstrual cycle is through activation of the hypothalamic-pituitary-adrenal (HPA) axis, which is similar to the reproductive hormonal axis (hypothalamic-pituitary-ovarian axis) we learned about on page xx. So, just as the hypothalamus regulates the release of sex hormones that play a key role in regulating your menstrual cycle, it also controls the release of stress hormones (and many other hormone systems in the body). When we experience significant stress, either physically (e.g., due to overexercising, lack of sleep or malnourishment) or psychologically (e.g., a stressful life event), the HPA axis kicks into action, causing the release of stress hormones. These stress hormones have multiple effects on the body, one of which is suppressing normal levels of reproductive hormones, which essentially leads to irregular cycles. This is how stress can drive period loss in the case of hypothalamic amenorrhea (HA) and why stress management is a key pillar in the management of this condition.

Think of it like this: the stress response is a protective mechanism to keep you safe. When it senses a threat, it relays to the body that right now is not a safe or healthy time to have a baby, so it deactivates those hormone systems.

In order to make the body feel safe, we need to make sure we are

Diagram to follow

nourished, cared for and well-rested, with adequate sleep, nutrition, a safe environment and a support system (partner/friend/family).

PMS/PMDD

Not all women will experience mood changes related to their menstrual cycle, but for those who do, it's typically in the days before the onset of the next period. There are over 150 different physical, psychological and behavioural symptoms that may occur premenstrually, from bloating and breast pain to mood swings and irritability. In a survey of over 40,000 women, the second most common premenstrual symptom, reported by 77 per cent of participants, were psychological symptoms, including low mood or irritability.[26] However, while most (80–90 per cent) menstruating women experience any combination of premenstrual symptoms during this time, a smaller, but still large, group of women experience symptoms so bad it interferes with their essential, basic self-care tasks and quality of life.[27] This is known as premenstrual syndrome (PMS), and affects approximately 20–40 per cent of women, while premenstrual dysphoric disorder (PMDD), which includes similar physical symptoms to PMS but with much more severe emotional and behavioural symptoms, is found in 2–8 per cent of women.[28] [29]

PMS and PMDD are both cyclical in nature, with symptoms starting in the luteal phase of the menstrual cycle (about 1–2 weeks before the period starts) and improving once the period begins, or shortly after. However, while they share a similar pattern, and can both have physical and emotional symptoms, PMS and PMDD are separate conditions and have notable differences. PMDD is a diagnostic mood disorder and can have a much greater negative impact on your daily activities and quality of life: it is estimated that that those with PMDD experience a total of 1,400 days or 3.835 years of disability adjusted life years (DALYs) lost due to the disorder.[30] In 2013, PMDD was listed as a depressive disorder in the *DSM-V*, a key manual doctors use to diagnose mental health issues, and in 2019 it was also added to the International Classification of Diseases, recognizing PMDD worldwide as a legitimate medical condition that requires diagnosis and treatment. As PMDD is chronic and recurring, it is also recognized as a disability under the Equality Act 2010. This means employers must make reasonable accommodations to assist employees with PMDD.

What causes PMS/PMDD?

As with many aspects related to female health, due to a lack of scientific research, we don't know exactly what causes PMS or PMDD, and why some women are affected and others are not. Compared to women who don't suffer from PMS, those who do have similar levels of hormones, but appear to be more sensitive to these hormonal fluctuations.[31] One hormone of particular interest in relation to PMDD is allopregnanolone, or 'allo', a byproduct of progesterone. Allo acts on the same receptors as alcohol and benzodiazepines (such as Xanax), producing anti-anxiety and sedative effects. In PMDD, it is believed that allo interacts with these receptors in a dysfunctional way, contributing to the mood-related symptoms seen in PMDD, such as irritability, mood swings and anxiety.[32] [33] Some, but not all, family and twin studies support a genetic component to PMS/PMDD.[34] [35] Ultimately, there are many ongoing areas of research into the causes of PMDD; it may be that PMDD results from a combination of hormonal, neurobiological and genetic factors.

Getting diagnosed

The diagnosis of PMS and PMDD is based on the timing of symptoms and their degree of impact on daily life. When seeking a diagnosis, it's helpful to keep a symptom diary for at least 2–3 cycles to document the symptoms and their relationship to your cycle. Your doctor may also ask you to complete a questionnaire. In the case of PMDD, at least 5 of the 11 symptoms listed below must be present, one of which must be a 'core symptom' (given in bold).

DIAGNOSTIC CRITERIA FOR PREMENSTRUAL DYSPHORIC DISORDER (PMDD)

---

1. Marked affective lability (e.g., mood swings, feeling suddenly sad or tearful, or increased sensitivity to rejection)

2. Marked irritability or anger or increased interpersonal conflicts

3. Marked depressed mood, feelings of hopelessness or self-deprecating thoughts

4. Marked anxiety, tension and/or feelings of being keyed up or on edge

5. Decreased interest in usual activities (e.g., work, school, friends, hobbies)

6. Subjective difficulty in concentration

7. Lethargy, easy fatiguability or marked lack of energy

8. Marked change in appetite; overeating; or specific food cravings

9. Hypersomnia (excessive sleepiness) or insomnia (trouble falling or staying asleep)

10. A sense of being overwhelmed or out of control

11. Physical symptoms such as breast tenderness or swelling, joint or muscle pain, a sensation of 'bloating', or weight gain

While there is no test to diagnose PMS or PMDD, blood tests will occasionally be ordered by your doctor to rule out other causes for symptoms. It's also important to rule out other disorders with overlapping symptoms, like depression and anxiety, which can also worsen premenstrually. This is known as premenstrual exacerbation (PME), and, unlike PMDD, symptoms are generally present throughout the entire cycle but can become more severe in the premenstrual phase.[36]

Unfortunately, getting diagnosed with PMS or PMDD is not always easy (or straightforward), and awareness of both conditions, in particular PMDD, is not very well known – even among health professionals. Taken from a paper of women's experiences of receiving a diagnosis, one said 'the [male] doctor that I saw told me that there was no such thing as PMDD, there was no such thing as PMS and this it is just something that women say'.[37]

Not only is this gaslighting women, but it creates barriers and delays to a diagnosis of PMDD, which when left untreated can evolve into secondary issues, including eating disorders, substance misuse problems and suicidal behaviour.[38] Devastatingly, 34 per cent of self-diagnosed PMDD sufferers have made a suicide attempt at some point in their lives. This is much higher than the general population, which is about 6 per cent in the UK.[39]

So, it's imperative that we raise awareness of PMDD and work to abolish the stigma attached to women presenting with menstruation-related concerns.

Case Study: Sophia

At 26 years old, Sophia was struggling to get a diagnosis of PMDD and endometriosis, and was beginning to accept that every month she would have not only pain and bloating the week of her period, but severe mood changes in the 7–10 days before. She explained to me how she feels she only has 'one good week of the month', because the week or two before her period she feels incredibly low in mood, more irritable and extremely fatigued. Her healthy habits of going to the gym and cooking nourishing meals often go out the window during this time and are swapped for days in bed and ordering takeout. Once her period arrives, she starts to feel better in mood, and by the end of her period she feels back to herself, her mood is lifted and her energy levels are high. This lasts for about a week or so before the cycle starts again. One of the first things I asked her to do was to start tracking her cycle and her mood symptoms. Her pattern in mood and energy was like clockwork, so we worked on preparing for this in her 'good weeks'. This meant batch cooking and preparing meals that could be put in the freezer for the 'less good week' (as we called it), scheduling in lower-impact forms of movement like a walk with a friend, making more time for self-care and prioritizing sleep.

While these changes did not 'cure' her PMDD, they allowed Sophia to better manage the impact of PMDD and endometriosis on her daily life. The structured approach helped her maintain some level of consistency in her self-care routines, even during the more difficult phases of her cycle. Over time, she described to me how she felt more in control of her symptoms and less overwhelmed by the monthly fluctuations in mood and energy.

Treatment for PMS and PMDD

Lifestyle

Lifestyle changes alone may be more appropriate for mild PMS than for PMDD, but are important for everyone in terms of supporting overall health.

Nutrition

There is no specific 'diet' that can be used to treat PMS or PMDD, but it is recommended to follow a healthy, balanced diet while limiting caffeine, alcohol and salt, all of which may exacerbate certain symptoms such as bloating, sleep disturbance and irritability. Often sugar (and carbs in general) get the blame for worsening symptoms in PMS/PMDD, but this link has not been demonstrated in the research.[40] [41] That said, while sugar may not *cause* PMS or PMDD, during this part of the cycle (the luteal phase), energy levels and blood sugar levels are less stable, so it would still be a smart idea to limit foods high in free sugars (such as cakes, sweets and chocolate), which give us fast but fleeting boosts in energy, for complex carbohydrates (found in wholegrains, pulses and veggies), which gives us sustained energy, alongside additional nutrients like fibre and B vitamins.

Supplements

The following supplements may help improve PMS and PMDD symptoms for some people, but the evidence is mixed, with some studies showing benefits, others not. There is also little data on how well these supplements work for the severe emotional symptoms of PMDD. As always, please make sure to discuss with your healthcare provider before starting any new supplements.

Chasteberry (Vitex agnus-castus)

Chasteberry has been shown to be effective in reducing PMS symptoms and physical symptoms of PMDD.[42] [43] [44] While it is generally well-tolerated, there is no standard recommended dose, and it is not suitable for people on certain medications, including antipsychotics like olanzapine, or those who are breastfeeding or pregnant. There is also some concern that it may decrease the effectiveness of oral contraceptives or hormone replacement therapy.

Calcium and vitamin D

Taking calcium carbonate (1,200 mg per day) has been shown to reduce PMS symptoms in clinical trials.[45] [46] However, another small study found that calcium supplementation was not any better than a placebo for PMDD.[47] Low levels of calcium and vitamin D during the second half of the menstrual cycle may worsen PMS symptoms. Conversely, women who eat diets high in vitamin D and calcium are less likely to develop PMS.[48] [49] Good sources of calcium and vitamin D are listed in the nutrition chapter on page xx.

Magnesium

Magnesium supplementation may also be helpful in reducing PMS symptoms, including mood changes and fluid retention.[50] [51] [52] One study looked at the effect of magnesium and vitamin B6 supplementation together, and results showed that when taken in combination, they had a greater effect on PMS management compared with taking magnesium alone.[53] It is important to note that these effects on PMS were shown after a few months of taking a supplement consistently. While these studies used supplements, magnesium can also be obtained through the diet, so, if symptoms are mild, that may be a good place to start. Good sources of magnesium include: nuts and seeds, leafy greens (such as spinach), kidney beans, wholewheat bread and brown rice.

Other Supplements

Despite limited evidence, vitamin B6 (pyridoxine) is often recommended for PMS.[54] However, some women find supplementation helpful. Please note that toxicity (including nerve damage) can occur with doses as low as 200mg/day, so recommended doses are 25–100mg/day.

Several other supplements, such as vitamin E, evening primrose oil and St John's Wort, are also often recommended for PMS, but there is not sufficient evidence to say whether they are more effective than not taking anything. If you wish to try these or other supplements, be sure to speak with your doctor about whether they are safe for you and how to use them.

Exercise

A recent review of 15 studies found that exercise can be an effective treatment for PMS, helping to ease psychological, physical and behavioural symptoms.[55] The best part? It doesn't matter which type of exercise you choose; what's important is finding something you love and sticking with it, as consistent, long-term exercise is key for the best outcome. It's natural and normal for your motivation and energy levels to fluctuate across your cycle – especially if you're someone who experiences PMS or PMDD – but even practicing yoga or going for a gentle walk can offer benefits.

Sleep

Women with PMS and PMDD are more likely to experience sleep problems like insomnia, especially during the late luteal phase leading up to the period. See page x for more information on optimizing sleep during this time. However, if your sleep problems are constant or chronic, it's essential to seek professional support.

Stress management

Often easier said than done, but stress reduction is an important part of managing your PMS and PMDD, as stress can exacerbate symptoms. I find stress reduction is quite personal and will look different to each individual, but some ideas might include: deep breathing exercises, meditation, taking a warm bath, listening to music, or yoga. If you find it hard to make time for these activities, try scheduling just 15 minutes of relaxation every day, especially in the luteal phase.

Medication, therapy and surgery

Beyond lifestyle changes, there are various treatment options available for PMS and PMDD, including:

* **Painkillers or anti-inflammatory drugs:** Non-steroidal anti-inflammatory drugs like ibuprofen can help with physical symptoms such as cramps and headaches.
* **Antidepressants:** Selective serotonin reuptake inhibitors (SSRIs) are a type of antidepressant which have been shown

to be effective for PMDD. They may be prescribed to be taken daily throughout the month or just during the luteal phase. Examples include fluoxetine and citalopram.

* **Hormonal contraception:** Some women find using the combined oral contraceptive pill helps with PMS/PMDD symptoms. Newer types of contraceptive pills containing a progestogen called Drospirenone have been shown to be particularly effective.[56] [57]

* **Cognitive-behavioural therapy (CBT):** This form of therapy focuses on changing negative thought patterns and behaviours and, in one clinical study, was found to be just as effective as antidepressants for managing PMDD.[58]

* **GnRH analogue injections (GnRH):** GnRH medications act on the pituitary gland in the brain to suppress ovulation and the production of ovarian hormones. It creates a temporary (and reversible) menopausal state, often referred to as 'chemical menopause'.

* **Surgery:** In very severe cases, where other treatment options have failed, your doctor might suggest considering a total hysterectomy (removal of the uterus) along with bilateral salpingo-oophorectomy (removal of the ovaries and fallopian tubes). The goal of this surgery is to help you find relief from PMDD symptoms by permanently stopping your monthly cycle.

Summary

* The link between the menstrual cycle and mental health is extremely complex, involving interactions between genetics, reproductive hormones and other physiological processes, as well as environmental factors, including lifestyle and social, political and structural influences on health and wellbeing.

* The link is also likely to be bidirectional: the menstrual cycle may influence our mental health, and psychological stress can impact the menstrual cycle, causing changes in flow and regularity, as well as loss of periods.

* Stress can downregulate reproductive hormones, leading to irregular periods or no periods at all.

* The majority of women experience premenstrual symptoms (90 per cent), a smaller percentage (20-40 per cent) experience premenstrual syndrome (PMS), whereby symptoms are so severe they interfere with daily life, and an even smaller percentage (3–8 per cent) experience premenstrual dysphoric disorder (PMDD), which includes similar physical symptoms to PMS but with much more severe emotional and behavioural symptoms.

Breast health

During my NHS years I did a lot of locum work for the breast surgery team, and as a result I've examined *a lot* of breasts over the years. I can tell you, therefore, that they come in all shapes and sizes; they can be lumpy or soft, hairy or asymmetrical, and they can change as we age and across the menstrual cycle. So, the most important thing when it comes to breast health is learning what *your* normal is – just like your cycle. Knowing what my normal was meant I was quick to find a breast lump a few years back and have it investigated at the One Stop breast clinic at my local hospital within two weeks. It turned out to be benign and not something to worry about – which is often the case with breast lumps. If you do find a lump, however, and it doesn't go, it's so incredibly important to speak to your GP. That said, breast cancer does not always present as a lump, and so looking out for other breast changes is equally important. So, let's take a look at the basics of breast anatomy . . .

Breast anatomy

The breasts are not just made up of fatty tissue covered by skin – oh no, they're pretty unique, and, I'm sure you will agree, pretty beautiful structures! Breast tissue is not only located in the breasts themselves, but extends from the boundaries of your clavicle, your breast bone/sternum, all the way into the armpit. This is why, when checking your breasts, or when being examined by a doctor, it's important not to forget the armpit and across the chest.

The breast is made up of three major components: connective (fibrous) tissue, glandular (mammary) tissue, and adipose (fat) tissue. The milk-producing glandular tissue is organized in lobules – and the lobules themselves are organized into around 15–20 lobes. Both the lobes and lobules are connected by milk ducts, which act as stems or tubes to carry the milk to the nipple. During pregnancy, the lobules grow and begin to produce milk.

The breast contains fibrous tissue known as Cooper's ligaments – but these are not 'true' ligaments, like the tough, flexible bands of connective tissue that connect bones to other bones in the body, and only provide limited support to the breasts (additional support is provided by the breast skin itself). The breasts also contain blood vessels, lymph vessels and nerves – for sensation.

Did you know? Breasts do not contain *any* muscle – but they do sit on top of the pectoral muscles (or the 'pecs') that are connected to the chest wall. So, any workout videos claiming to (and I quote) 'firm up saggy breasts' are unfortunately a waste of your time.

Lymph vessels and lymph nodes

You might have come across the term 'lymphatic drainage' used in therapeutic or aromatherapy massage, or perhaps you have heard about lymph nodes in relation to cancer, but, other than that, the lymphatic system is rarely spoken about. Essentially, that lymphatic system is part of the immune system and is made up lymph vessels, nodes and certain organs in the body. Its primary role is to help defend the body against infection and disease. The lymph vessels are similar to the arteries and veins in the body that carry blood, but they are much finer and carry a colourless liquid called lymph that contains white blood cells (important for immune defence). These vessels connect to groups of small lymph nodes throughout the body. The system also includes organs like the spleen and thymus that monitor the blood and detect and respond to harmful microorganisms and malignant cells. Close to the breast, there is a collection of nodes under the armpit called axillary lymph nodes. If breast cancer spreads outside of the breast, it usually goes here. However, you may feel an enlarged node when fighting a viral infection or after getting a vaccine. There are also lymph nodes near the breastbone and above the collarbone.

Nipples

The nipple contains several openings allowing for milk to flow through during lactation. However, the purpose of the nipple isn't just for delivering milk during breastfeeding – it also plays a role in sexual pleasure and arousal. In fact, for some, nipple stimulation can even induce orgasm. Nipples can become erect when aroused but also when cold, touched, during pregnancy and breastfeeding – and also due to your menstrual cycle (especially around ovulation).

The nipple is surrounded by slightly darker skin called the areola, which often has small little bumps (similar to goosebumps) which are called Montgomery tubercles or glands. They are usually more prominent during pregnancy and breastfeeding, and at different times in the menstrual cycle. You might also notice a few sparse hairs around your nipple area, which is totally normal too. A small percentage of people have inverted nipples (they point inwards rather than outwards and can appear like slits), which is normal, though if you find your nipple suddenly becomes inverted or changes in appearance or shape unexpectedly, it could be a sign

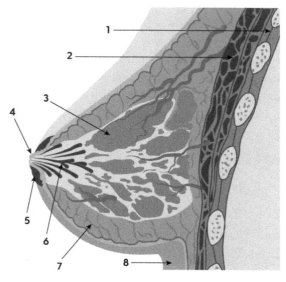

1 Chest wall
2 Pectoralis muscles
3 Lobules
4 Nipples
5 Areola
6 Milk duct
7 Fatty tissue
8 Skin

Structure of the female breast, adapted from: Love, S. M., Lindsey, K. (2015). *Dr. Susan Love's Breast Book.* United States: Hachette Books.[1]

of an underlying health condition and should be discussed with a health professional.

HEY IT'S OKAY IF . . .

---

* One breast is slightly bigger than the other – 94 per cent of women naturally have uneven breasts.[2]

* You have a few hairs around your nipple – the skin around the areolas contains hair follicles. Some people have fair hairs; some people have dark hairs.

* Your nipples point up, down, inwards or lay flat – not all nipples point straight ahead!

* You have stretch marks on your breast tissue – not everyone will get stretch marks on their breast, but it's very common as

breasts develop in puberty, during pregnancy or if your weight changes.

Note: While all of the above are variations of normal, if you suddenly notice changes to your breasts or nipples, or they change in size, it's important to get them checked out.

Breast changes across the menstrual cycle

'I usually get sore breasts the week before my period starts. There doesn't seem to be a pattern. Sometimes it's a few days of pain up to ten days before my period starts, and sometimes it's just a day or two before. Any pressure to my breasts hurts, and running or jumping is uncomfortable. They tend to swell the week before, too.' – **Raahki, 26**

Anyone who experiences a menstrual cycle will know that your breasts can change throughout the month, be that in size or tenderness. I often joke that I wish I had the shape and fullness of my premenstrual breasts all cycle long, but without the breast pain. In fact, my partner can often tell where I am at in my cycle based on my breasts alone, which some people may think is weird, but I think it's pretty great how well he knows my body and that we can have open discussions about normal bodily changes like this.

Just like the endometrium undergoes changes across the menstrual cycle, so does the breast tissue.[3] These changes are driven by fluctuations in levels of oestrogen, which causes breast ducts to grow in size, while progesterone promotes the growth of milk-producing glandular tissue and fluid retention within the breast tissue.

* At the start of the menstrual cycle, breasts are often less full, due to low levels of oestrogen and progesterone, with the volume of the breast at its lowest just after menstruation, between days 6 and 15.[4] [5]
* As the cycle progresses, particularly during the ovulatory phase, rising oestrogen levels can cause the breast ducts to enlarge, leading to increased breast size and tenderness.[6]
* Between around days 16 and 28, breast volume and water content increase, peaking after day 25.[7]
* After ovulation, progesterone production from the corpus luteum – a temporary structure in the ovary that forms after the egg is released – stimulates the growth of milk glands, which can make breasts feel fuller, tender and have a lumpy, 'cobblestone' texture. Breast volume increases up to 40 per cent the week before menstruation.[8]
* If pregnancy does not occur, oestrogen and progesterone levels drop, and breasts typically return to their preovulatory state, with reduced fullness and tenderness as the cycle ends and menstruation begins. *Note: It is not advisable to check your breasts during this time and it should be done after your period ends.*

Breast changes and hormonal contraception

Hormonal contraceptives can for some cause temporary changes such as increased breast tenderness or enlargement. In fact, one of the most common side effects for all contraception methods, as reported by the contraception review platform The Lowdown, is tender and enlarged breasts.[9] Certain methods are more commonly associated with this side effect; for example, users of the contraceptive patch report more breast discomfort, and it's often a reason to discontinue compared to pill users.[10] It can also happen with the hormonal IUD, but symptoms are often mild and resolve as the body adjusts to the hormones.[11] The good news is that these changes to the breast seem to be temporary. In studies comparing those who used combined oral contraceptives (COCs) or a hormonal IUD, there was no increase in breast density compared to those who never used hormonal contraceptives on mammogram scans. However, initially starting the pill was associated with an increase in breast density, suggesting that starting these contraceptives might temporarily affect breast density.[12] However, if your breasts feel uncomfortable and this persists after a few months of starting contraception, speak to a healthcare professional about your options.

For information on contraception and breast cancer risk, head back to page x.

Cyclical breast pain

If you find that your breasts are sore or uncomfortable in the days or weeks leading up to your period, and this is something that occurs monthly, you may have cyclical breast pain.

Cyclical pain is related to the menstrual cycle and affects up to two-thirds of women, with 1 in 10 women having moderate-to-severe pain.[13] It usually starts during the luteal phase of the cycle, within 2 weeks before the next period, and increases until the period begins and improves once it ends. The pain can occur anywhere, but is often described in the upper outer part of the breasts and can move to the underarm. The pain is also typically in both breasts, but the severity might be greater in one. Pain isn't the only downside, however, as cyclical breast pain can interfere with sexual activity (in 48 per cent of women), physical activity (37 per cent) and social (12 per cent), work or school (8 per cent) activity.[14]

In terms of treatment, for about 20–30 per cent of women it will resolve by itself, but unfortunately it can reoccur in the next couple of years.[15]

Tips to manage cyclical breast pain:

* In the first instance, make sure to wear a well-fitted bra during the day, for exercise, and a soft support bra at night.

* Topical anti-inflammatory medications, like ibuprofen gel, can reduce pain, as can simple painkillers such as paracetamol.[16] [17]

* Supplementation:

  • Evening primrose oil and vitamin E may improve symptoms in some women, though evidence is very limited and results have been inconsistent.[18] [19]

  • *Vitex agnus-castus* (also known as chasteberry) is another herbal treatment often used for menstrual-related breast pain.[20] [21] While it seems to be well-tolerated, it may interact with certain medications including antipsychotics and hormonal contraception and is not recommended in pregnancy, when breastfeeding or in those under 18 years of age.[22]

  • Flaxseed powder has shown to help with the duration and severity of cyclical breast pain.[23] [24] That said, in these studies participants consumed 25–30g of flaxseed powder, which equates to 5–6 tablespoons. High amounts of flaxseed can cause gut effects such as bloating, gas, pain, constipation and diarrhoea, so if you do choose to add more to your diet, make sure you slowly build up your tolerance and consume a lot of water alongside it.

* Hormonal contraception may sometimes be prescribed as a treatment for cyclical breast pain. However, breast pain can also be a side effect of hormonal contraception. Unfortunately, there's no real way to tell whether one or the other is likely to give you breast pain until you've tried it.

* Specialist treatment options are available if other methods don't work.

Note: It is always best to check with your pharmacist or doctor before taking any new supplements, to make sure that they don't interact with any other medications you may be taking or impact a health condition you may have.

Note: Breast pain is not always cyclical or related to the menstrual cycle. If you're experiencing pain, be that intermittent or constant, and it's ongoing, it's best to keep a symptom diary and speak to your doctor.

Breasts and exercise

Over 72 per cent of women who exercise report exercise-induced breast pain.[25] [26] While the exact source of the pain is not yet clear, studies have linked it to the movement of the breasts – and not just up and down, but also side to side, and forwards and backwards.[27] A statistic which *shocked* me is that unsupported breasts move 1cm vertically while we walk, up to 15cm during running, and almost 19cm during a jumping jack.[28] [29] [30] If left unsupported, this repetitive motion can strain and stretch the Coopers ligaments, the relatively weak connective tissue within the breast. The amount of movement and breast pain increases with the type of exercise (i.e., low vs high intensity exercise) and also the size of the breast. In fact, women with large breasts are less likely to take part in vigorous exercise, report increased pressure and pain from shoulder straps (which can also cause arm tingling and numbness due to nerve compression), more frictional injuries from sports bras, and greater difficulty finding the correct bra fit, than smaller-breasted women.[31]

Even if you have itty-bitty breasts, however, I want you to keep reading and listen to what I have to say next, as not only can lack of breast support lead to breast pain, breast ptosis (or 'sag'), and cause embarrassment for women, but all of these factors ultimately prevent women and girls from taking part in exercise and sport – which has a huge knock-on effect on overall health. In fact, one study reported that 17 per cent of women consider their breasts a barrier to exercise, but, in the same study, those who reported greater breast health knowledge were more likely to participate in sport and exercise. So, by informing and empowering women, we can help improve physical activity levels.[32] Likewise, 46 per cent of girls (aged 11–18) avoid physical activity because of their breasts, and over 50 per cent have never worn a sports bra. Within this study almost 90 per cent of girls wanted to know more about their breasts, highlighting a huge educational opportunity.[33] Teachers, parents and healthcare providers of teenage girls, I urge you to start the conversation around breast health soon. (Check out TreasureYourChest.Org for breast education resources and lesson plans.)

If I've yet to convince you to care about your sports bra, what if I told you that your choice of support can impact your performance, including how efficiently you run and even how you breathe?[34] And it makes sense, right? One of the cardinal signs of a pain or an injury is immobilization, after all. For example, if you hurt your leg, you will limp to reduce the amount of pain you experience. If your breasts start to cause discomfort when you run, you're going to (likely subconsciously) change how you run and how you breathe to try to reduce breast bounce and offset some of that pain. Personally, I avoid my hardest and longest runs in the days leading up to my period when my breasts are most tender – and you will never find me doing a burpee during this time either.

Once again, as with most aspects related to women's health, research into whether breasts can negatively affect performance is in its infancy, but one study investigating breast mass on marathon performance found that women with larger breasts had completed fewer marathons and had slower marathon finish times compared to smaller-breasted runners (there was a difference of approximately 35 minutes between a woman with 36A breast size to a woman with 36DD breast size). Some – but not all – of this difference can be explained by a higher BMI in larger-breasted women.[35] Ultimately, your breasts could be slowing down your pace and putting you at a disadvantage in races, so how much of a difference can a sports bra make? Well, another small study of 10 women (breast size 32DD or 34D) looked at the difference between wearing a low-impact sports bra vs. a high-impact sports bra on a 5km treadmill run (speed consistent for each). The researchers found that when wearing the high-impact sports bra, women had better running economy and form, suggesting that with the right support, you could potentially become a better runner.[36]

Breast awareness

Over the years, there has been some debate over just how valuable breast self-examination is in detecting breast cancer early and reducing deaths from breast cancer.[37] Because of the ongoing uncertainty raised by some studies, some organizations such as the American Cancer Society no longer recommend regular breast self-exams as a screening tool for women who do not have a high risk of breast cancer. This is because the risk and consequences of over-treating benign or normal lumps may outweigh the benefits of early detection. However, they do encourage women to be breast aware and know what is normal for them. In the UK, we are still encouraging women to get to know their normal and to check themselves regularly. Some people like to pop a monthly reminder in their phone, or remember to 'feel on the first', but it's generally best to check about 2-3 days after your period has ended, when your breasts are less lumpy. Breast cancer can affect all people, of all genders, so it's important that everyone is body aware.

How to check your breasts

* **LOOK:** Stand in front of the mirror with your hands on your hips. Scan your breasts for any changes. Raise your hands

above your head and have another look, and then another with your hands on your hips pushing inwards to tense your muscles.

* **FEEL:** Feel each breast. This can be done standing up or lying down. Examine each breast with the opposite hand and place your free arm behind your head. Using a flat hand, gently check one breast at a time using a systematic approach – quadrants is an easy way to do it. Don't forget to feel all the way up to the collarbones and into the armpits.

Things to look and feel for:

* Changes in skin colour
* Obvious lumps
* Changes in texture such as puckering or dimpling (like the skin of an orange)
* Redness or a rash on the skin and/or around the nipple
* Changes to the nipple (inversion or change in direction)
* Nipple discharge
* Unusual change in size or shape of the breast
* Any lumps in the breast, armpit or around the collarbones
* Thickening of the skin
* Discomfort or pain in one breast that is new and doesn't go away (Breast pain is a rare symptom of breast cancer, but new-onset pain should be assessed)

Found something unusual or concerning? Don't panic – for most people these changes will not be serious. Even so, it's still important to make an appointment with your GP as soon as possible.

Summary

* The breast is made up of three major components: connective (fibrous) tissue, glandular (mammary) tissue and adipose (fat) tissue.

* Breasts can change throughout the menstrual cycle in size, firmness, texture and tenderness.

* Many women have breast pain as part of their menstrual cycle. This is called cyclical breast pain.

* Hormonal contraceptives can for some cause temporary changes such as increased breast tenderness or enlargement.

* Unsupported breasts during exercise can lead to pain and impaired performance.

* When checking your breasts, it is best to do so 2–3 days after the period has ended, when your breasts are less lumpy.

Body image

Within magazines, social media, TV shows and movies, women are constantly bombarded with messages regarding how their body 'should' look in order to be considered beautiful and accepted – and while beauty is claimed to be in the eye of the beholder, in the media of Western society, beauty is usually reduced to one ideal body type: thin, toned, white, and often filtered. This pressure can cause many women to control and discipline themselves through extreme diets and back-to-back peloton classes, all to achieve this unrealistic (and often physiologically unattainable) body type. I see it all the time in my clinic, in my DMs, and when I scroll through TikTok, where women cut their calories to that of a toddler and spend a small fortune on reformer Pilates classes to have a flatter stomach or thinner arms. Yet this so-called 'ideal' body type is not always representative of a sustainable, healthy body. We're all built differently, and for many girls and women, this body type is simply unattainable. The disconnect caused by the 'ideal' vs the reality often leads to body concerns and poor body image, increasing the risk of depression, low self-esteem and eating disorders.[1] [2]

However, the media is not the only thing that impacts our body image; our peers and our family also have a role to play. For example, if you grew up in a household where your parents often spoke negatively about their own bodies or other people's bodies,[3] [4] or relatives made off-hand comments about your appearance, you are more likely to be unhappy with your body in adulthood.[5] [6] [7] One comment may not seem hugely impactful in isolation, but over time, they can have pretty negative and long-lasting cumulative effects. I acutely remember a family friend once commenting on the 'freshers fifteen' weight I had gained after my first year in university, and feeling utterly mortified and deeply ashamed of myself. It stuck with me, and I started my first diet the very next day.

Conversely, children of parents who are more self-compassionate and speak positively about their bodies tend to have higher body self-esteem and engage in less emotional eating.[8] When I learned this, I stopped engaging in 'fat talk' with other women – you know, where we go back and forth sharing our body insecurities, like 'I hate my thighs' or 'look at my muffin top'. Yeah, that. I used to do it to fit in and make friends, but I've come to realize it's a useless (and toxic) way of bonding and it made me more unhappy in my body. What I've learned over time, and what is reflected in the research, is that women prefer other women who engage in positive body talk.[9] When you stop and think about it, the best and most memorable conversations you've had with your friends probably had nothing to do with calories or bodyweight. Nowadays, I like to share non-body related thoughts or comments with my girlfriends, such as about a book I'm currently loving or a trip I'm planning to take, instead of the methods I'm using to try to shrink my body or how 'naughty' I was by having dessert last night.

In addition to how people around us speak about their bodies and the pressure imposed on us by the media to attain unrealistic body standards, the menstrual cycle can also influence body image. Personally, you cake it as a signal I'm premenstrual if you see me in the gym in an oversized hoodie and a pair of leggings – partly for comfort, but also to focus less attention on my body. The relationship between body image and the menstrual cycle is complex, and while our bodies may only physically change temporarily and only in a small way, how we perceive ourselves can fluctuate quite significantly. Let's explore how.

'Body image' is a term that can be used to describe how we think, feel and act with regard to our body.[10] 'Body image concerns' refer to feelings of being unsatisfied with our body – either because of its appearance, shape/weight, or the way it functions. This is also described as 'body dissatisfaction'.

There are four components of body image:

1. Cognitive – the thoughts and beliefs that you hold about your body

2. Behavioural – how you behave as a result of your body image

3. Perceptual – how you see/perceive yourself

4. Affective – how you feel about your body

Body image and the menstrual cycle

Around ovulation, many women report feeling more physically attractive, compared to the luteal phase, and are less likely to focus on parts of their body they deem 'unattractive'.[11] [12] [13] One study reported changes in clothing preferences where women were more likely to choose clothing that is more revealing and 'sexy' around ovulation.[14] While these changes are subtle, it's thought that they are due to evolutionary factors and increased social and sexual confidence during this time in the menstrual cycle.

In the luteal phase, just before the next period, we may have a tendency to be more self-critical and feel more uncomfortable in our bodies.[15] Interestingly, in one study they found body dissatisfaction was highest during the period, but there were no significant changes to anthropomorphic (body) measurements.

This essentially means that we believe we look different or bigger, but our bodies haven't physically changed significantly – which is why it's so important to develop positive body image.[16] That said, some women do often gain weight physically (from retaining water) around this time, which can also influence body image.

Premenstrual symptoms such as bloating (which tends to be worse on day 1 of menstruation and decreases as the cycle progresses[17] [18]) and breast tenderness can also affect how women perceive their bodies. Mood changes and emotional symptoms during the luteal phase can also contribute to a more critical body image. In fact, body dissatisfaction is particularly heightened in women with PMS. In research interviews with women who have premenstrual disorders (such as PMS and PMDD), many of them described their premenstrual bodies as 'fat', 'ugly', 'unattractive' or compared them to animals such as 'whale' and 'elephant'.[19] Some of these negative feelings were associated with physical changes, such as bloating and painful breasts, but women also described themselves as more 'self-conscious' and 'self-critical' of their bodies during this part of the cycle.[20] So it seems that, while our bodies may change a little, we are also more likely to pick ourselves apart.

'Every single month, without fail, a few days before my period, I will text one of my friends (because she had a similar thing) and I'm like, I hate my body, every time. And I'm like, I don't actually. I quite like my body, but without fail, I will feel awful about myself. I talk to myself in the worst way.' – **Lily, 27**

For many women, premenstrual cravings and the out-of-control feeling around food during this time can make them feel worse, and also play a role in premenstrual distress and body dissatis-faction.[21] Which just highlights the clutches that diet culture and the pursuit of thinness have on us; we can't even relax when we're feeling rubbish, at least not without feeling guilty and engaging in compensatory behaviours the following week.

The good news is, not everyone experiences negative body image before or during menstruation, and even if you do, by working on our relationship with our bodies (more on this next) and improving our body image, we're more likely to have a better experience of our menstrual cycles too.[22]

The pill and body image

We don't know as much about how hormonal contraception affects body image, but one study found that while body image didn't change much throughout the menstrual cycle, people on hormonal contraception tended to focus more on the parts of their body they liked the least,[23] and in another, women report-ing a history of oral contraceptive side effects had higher levels of body dissatisfaction, even when we take body mass index (BMI) into account.[24] Another factor to consider is potential weight gain, which is often something women are concerned about when it comes to the pill and their body image. However, a review of 49 trials of pills and patches found that most studies showed no large weight difference.[25] Overall, there is no real con-clusive evidence, and more research is needed to understand how hormonal contraception can impact body image and body weight.

Improving body image

Building a positive body image takes time, and it doesn't mean you will always be happy with your body. The aim is to get to a point where we can experience thoughts or feelings about our bodies without the need to act on them or change them. Beyond having a better relationship with your body and your menstrual cycle, positive body image is associated with:

* Higher self-esteem
* Lower depression scores
* Healthier diet behaviours and patterns
* Improved feelings of wellbeing[26]

With that in mind, here are some tips on how to improve your own body image:

1. Focus on functionality

Focusing on everything your body can *do* – rather than how it *looks* – has been linked to more positive body image and greater engagement in physical activity.[27] Conversely, women who exercise for appearance-related reasons, such as to burn more calories or get a flatter stomach, are more likely to experience eating disorder symptoms (such as negative feelings towards the body), as well as higher symptoms of depression and lower self-esteem.[28] Similarly, in teenage girls, body appearance-related pride (i.e., 'I am proud of how good my body looks') is negatively related to levels of activity, while body fitness-related pride (i.e., 'I am proud of how strong my body is') is positively associated.[29] Essentially, focusing on what the body can do is linked to higher activity levels, while placing too much emphasis on appearance may be associated with less engagement in physical activity. When setting health goals, perhaps consider how you can base the goal around performance over appearance, e.g., running your first half marathon as opposed to running to earn dessert later. Not only will this improve your body image, but it will make exercise a lot more enjoyable!

2. Spring-clean your social media feed

Social media isn't inherently bad, and in some situations can be a platform for body positivity and inspiration for health and performance goals. However, there's no denying it can also contribute to unrealistic beauty standards and unhealthy comparisons. The more we compare how we look to people we follow on social media, the more we increase our body dissatisfaction.[30][31] Even #fitspiration or #fitspo content, while potentially well-intended, can negatively impact body image and mental health, as it promotes exercise for weight loss and appearance-based reasons.[32] If you use social media, I'd urge you to reflect on how the accounts you follow make you feel about yourself and perhaps consider unfollowing (or muting) accounts that may trigger unhelpful thoughts about your body. Instead, seek out accounts with more diverse bodies and also accounts that are unrelated to fitness (who doesn't love a good food page?!). The more you do this, the less the algorithms will push this type of content to you, and over time your feed will be a less triggering place. If and when bad body image days do happen (perhaps around menstruation), this might be a good time to take a day or two offline and focus your attention on things that make you feel good, like spending time with your loved ones, getting lost in a book or new TV series, or cooking your favourite meal.

3. Practice body gratitude and appreciation

Sometimes the 'just love your body' message can feel like a pretty seismic jump, but perhaps a good place to start is working toward body appreciation. This isn't always easy to do because we are not programmed to celebrate our bodies and all they do for us. As with any new skill, it might feel a bit uncomfortable in the beginning, but with practice will become easier.

Some prompts to consider might be:

- How does my body allow me to do my favourite activities? (e.g., dancing, playing with your kids, painting, travelling . . .)
- What do I appreciate about what my body has done for me today/this week/lately? (related to the menstrual cycle, this might be how your womb sheds, repairs and rebuilds every month!)
- What amazing experience have I had because of my body? (e.g., giving birth, running a 10k, dancing at your best friend's wedding)

4. Consider the conversations you're having with yourself and others

When talking or thinking about ourselves – or speaking to others – try to avoid engaging in unhelpful 'fat talk'. Of course, your best mates should be the people you can confide in about your insecurities, and vice versa, but that's a little different to tearing yourself down constantly or basing your conversations with them solely around your body/appearance, diets and weight loss. If you find that in your friendship circle these topics keep popping up, consider setting boundaries by saying something along the lines of, 'Talking about weight, physical appearance and body size isn't helpful for me. Can we talk about something else when we hang out?' If that feels too confronting for you, try changing the conversation with a pivot like 'I've been hoping to chat to you about . . .' Remember, the most interesting thing about you is not your body or clothes size, but who you are as a person.

Summary

* Body image is a term that can be used to describe how we think, feel and act with regard to our bodies.

* Body image is influenced by many different aspects, including family, peers, partners, the media and the menstrual cycle.

* Body image concerns are greater during the premenstrual and menstrual phases.

* More research is needed to understand how hormonal contraception can impact body image and body weight.

* By working on improving our body image, we're more likely to have a better experience of our menstrual cycles.

Sex and libido

Whether you've noticed a pattern or not, it's perfectly normal for your interest in sex to fluctuate throughout your monthly cycle.

Sexual desire (or libido as it is commonly known) is having an interest in engaging in sexual activity. A high level of desire simply means you want sex a lot – but it's not constant, and can ebb and flow depending on several variables such as age, health, relationships and the menstrual cycle. Conditions such as PCOS can also have an effect on sexual desire and reduce sexual satisfaction.[1]

It is important to note, however, that the same things can affect different people in different ways. For example, while some may find that work stress is a passion killer, others may use it as a way to relax after a stressful week. Similarly, while there are certain points in the menstrual cycle where women typically report increased desire and arousal, we're not machines, and there are many other factors that impact our interest, or lack thereof, in having sex (e.g., looming deadlines or in-laws coming to visit).

Sexual desire and the menstrual cycle

In general, it's been shown in the research that sex drive is highest at points in the menstrual cycle when progesterone is low and oestrogen levels are high (i.e., around ovulation).

One study collected hormone levels across 1–2 menstrual cycles from a group of naturally cycling women (i.e., not on contraception) alongside diary reports of their sexual behaviour (whether or not they had sex or masturbated) and subjective sexual desire (e.g., how much they wanted sex).[2] They found there was a mid-cycle peak in sexual desire when oestrogen is high, around ovulation, and it makes sense, right? From an evolutionary point of view, it's prime baby-making time! Whereas, after ovulation, in the luteal phase, when progesterone is high, there was a fall in sexual desire (see image below).

Diagram to follow

Adapted from: Roney JR, Simmons ZL. Hormonal predictors of sexual motivation in natural menstrual cycles. Hormones and Behavior, 2013 Apr 1;63(4):636–45.[3]

Interestingly, sexual desire may vary depending on whether or not you experience premenstrual symptoms. One small study found that those with premenstrual symptoms reported a peak in sexual interest around ovulation, but those without premenstrual symptoms reported a peak premenstrually (before the next period!).[4] I found this incredibly interesting (as someone who is absolutely not *in the mood* before my period), but I guess at this point in the cycle, your progesterone levels drop, which could positively impact libido.

> *'I have zero libido in the run-up to my cycle and during it. This also ties in with lower emotional connection, as I find myself feeling extremely irritable and the mood swings affect how keen I am for connection. During ovulation, my libido increases and I feel more connected to my partner.'* – **Zoe, 36**

Despite the various anecdotes and theories proposed about how the menstrual cycle impacts sexual desire, the results are inconclusive and, in some cases, contradictory. Much of the research on menstrual cycle-related changes in sexual desire also ignores how physical and psychological changes of the menstrual cycle (e.g., cramps, nausea, mood swings) might impact sexual desire. A recent study aimed to explore this by asking female university students to complete a daily questionnaire on their sexual desire, psychological changes and physical changes over the course of two menstrual cycles. Similar to previous research, they found that the menstrual cycle was indeed associated with a small mid-cycle increase in sexual desire, but there was a large variation in their results. Specifically, some reported a increase before their period, and some had no change in sexual desire across the menstrual cycle.[5] Arguably the most interesting finding was that happiness was the strongest predictor of change in sexual desire (i.e., increasing sexual desire) among all of the measured physical and psychological changes. Things like depressed mood, mood swings, low energy and back/join point were all associated with decreased sexual desire.

To sum up: the menstrual cycle does not impact the sexual desire of all women in the same way, and while it has an influence, it's not the *only* influence. In my opinion, it's better not to assume women are (or are not) interested in sex based on where they're at in their cycle, because not only does it oversimply something which is quite complex and multifaceted, but it can add unnecessary pressure on a woman, be that self-inflicted or within relationships.

Sexual desire and the pill

Women on hormonal contraception are unlikely to experience the same fluctuations in their libido. While some women may not notice any changes to their sex drive while taking the pill, some say it goes up and others will say it goes down. In a 2013 review of the few studies available, looking at the pill and sexual desire, most women reported no change in libido, a smaller number noticed an increase, and an even smaller number reported a decrease.[6] The formulation and regimen of the hormonal contraception seems to matter too, as the researchers found that women using pills with the smallest dose of oestrogen available reported having a decreased libido, while those using pills with higher doses of oestrogen generally experienced no change or an increase in libido.[7] Another study compared how women taking the pill differed, sexually, from people using a placebo in seven areas of sexual function.[8] Both participants and the researchers were unaware who got the active drug (in this case the pill) or the placebo, which reduces the risk of bias.[9] After 3 months of treatment, they found that women in the pill group were more likely to report decreased sexual desire, arousal and pleasure – but this did not seem to mean they had less sex, or less good sex. Both groups reported about the same number of 'satisfying sexual episodes' and the same scores for questions about orgasm.[10]

Regardless of what the research says, one of the key predictors of women discontinuing or switching pills is the sexual side effects.[11] When deciding whether to start, continue or stop a form of contraception, it's important to think about what makes a good sexual experience for you and – of course – weigh up all of the other risks and benefits with your doctor.

Can orgasm help with period pain?

Having sex or masturbating during menstruation is not everyone's bag, and granted it can be quite messy, but for those who are up for a bit of period sex, it can actually act as a natural pain reliever.

While sex on your period is still a pretty taboo topic, theoretically it could help with period pain. During and after orgasm, certain hormones are released that impact the body in positive ways. These hormones include endorphins, oxytocin and dopamine. Endorphins have a direct impact on the perception and processing of pain and counteract the effect of prostaglandins (which are thought to be responsible for period pain, see page XX). As well as reducing pain, oxytocin also reduces the stress hormone cortisol, and dopamine is a hormone that is responsible for feelings of pleasure, desire and motivation. At the same time, blood flow is increased to the area, which can have a relaxing effect on the muscles. There are no clinical studies looking specifically at the impact of orgasm as a result of sexual intercourse on period pain, but there is an interesting study done by Lunette, a menstrual cup brand, and Womanizer, a (terribly named) sex toy brand. In this study, aptly named 'Menstrubation', a total of 486 people were asked to forgo their traditional methods of pain control over the course of 3 months and to masturbate instead. 70 per cent said that regular masturbation made an impact on the intensity of their period pain, and 62 per cent said it made an impact on the frequency. When it comes to period-pain relief, 43 per cent of the participants thought medication was more effective, while 42 per cent said masturbation and the remaining 15 per cent preferred a mix of both, or other methods such as heat, CBD (cannabidiol), exercise and sleep.[12] Now, this research has a lot of limitations, and is riddled with bias, but those numbers are still impressive. When it comes to alternative therapies, it's helpful to ask yourself: can this do me any harm? And if the answer is no, and at worst it's a waste of your time, then perhaps it's worth trying, if only as an adjuvant to your usual pain relief.

Summary

* Sexual desire (or libido) is having an interest in engaging in sexual activity.

* Some women experience changes to desire and arousal across the menstrual cycle. This is in part due to hormones, but also a result of physical and psychological symptoms related to the menstrual cycle.

* While some women may not notice any changes to their sex drive while taking the pill, some report a decrease and others an increase. However, one of the main reasons women discontinue or switch pills is due to sexual side effects.

* Sex and masturbation may help with period pain.

Skin and hair

I doubt it's news to you that hormones can affect our skin – anyone who has gone through puberty can attest to that. It's the awkward reality of being a teenager: not only do you have to deal with, let's be honest, quite significant changes to your body, but your skin goes through the ringer, too, and no one really prepares you for that. The truth is, it doesn't just stop at puberty, and hormonal fluctuations across the menstrual cycle can bring you through a full spectrum of skin changes in just one month, from glowing, hydrated skin to unruly breakouts. For many, the unwelcome arrival of a huge, throbbing, has-its-own-heartbeat kind of spot is often the first warning sign that their period is just around the corner. And consider yourself lucky if this is isolated to one spot, because for about half of women, this constitutes a premenstrual flare of hormonal acne which can be incredibly painful, inflamed and very tricky to get a handle on.[1] The good news is that understanding how your skin responds to different phases of your cycle means you can implement preventative skincare tweaks to help offset those hormonal changes.

As hormone levels shift, skin conditions like eczema, psoriasis and rosacea can also flare up across the menstrual cycle. In one study, nearly half of all patients with eczema reported a deterioration in their condition in the week before their period which settles once their period starts.[2] The skin barrier becomes more permeable during this time, meaning it is more susceptible to the effects of both environmental allergens and general irritants, which likely explains why these flare-ups happen.[3]

Skin changes, like acne, can also be a sign of an underlying hormonal imbalance such as PCOS. I was pretty shocked to see a return in my acne aged 28, after years of clear skin, and what I didn't realize at the time was this was one of the first symptoms of PCOS that I experienced. In fact, my dermatologist suggested I speak to my doctor after she examined my skin and noted the hair thinning I was experiencing – another sign of PCOS. We'll chat more about this later in the chapter, and what we can do to help, but first, to understand how hormones impact our skin, it's important to understand its structure.

The skin structure

The skin is composed of three layers:

1. The epidermis
2. The dermis
3. The subcutaneous layer

The epidermis

The epidermis is the very top layer of skin, and the part we can see, but it's also the thinnest. In some parts of the body, the epidermis is thinner than others, like the epidermis around your eyes compared to the skin on your back.

The outer portion of the epidermis forms our skin barrier and protects us against UV radiation and harmful bacteria and viruses. It also retains moisture to prevent the skin from drying out. Still, it can become easily compromised by too much sun exposure or frequent use of strong active skincare products causing it to become dry, flaky and irritated. (Note to self: *If you look after your skin barrier, it will look after you.*)

Most of the cells in the epidermis are keratinocytes, which, as you might have guessed from the name, contain a protein called keratin, which helps to give our skin, hair and nails structure and strength. These keratinocyte cells come from deep in the epidermis and travel up to the surface where they are gradually shed and then replaced by newer cells pushed up from below. This entire renewal process takes an average of 28 days and is known as a skin 'cycle'. As we get older, the skin cycle slows down and takes longer, which leads to the accumulation of dead skin cells on the surface of the epidermis and loss of moisture overall, leaving the skin appearing dull and less firm. Regular exfoliation can help remove dead skin cells from the surface and improve skin texture and appearance, but it's worth remembering that over-exfoliation can cause more harm than good to the skin barrier.

There are also some other cells in the epidermis that produce the pigment melanin, aptly named melanocytes. The role of melanin is to protect against UV radiation from sunlight, which damages DNA and, over time, can lead to skin cancer. Melanin also contributes to our skin and hair colour – and the colour of our eyes.

Two other important cells that can be found in the epidermis are Langerhans cells, which form part of the immune system, and Merkel cells, which sense touch.

The dermis

The middle, and thickest, layer of the skin is the dermis. It is mostly fibrous, consisting of collagen and elastic fibres, and provides strength and elasticity. It also houses a whole host of appendages, such as blood vessels, lymph vessels, hair follicles, sebaceous (oil) glands, sensory neurons and cells such as

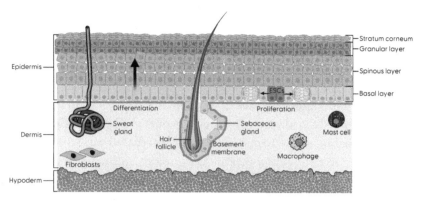

Adapted from: Gratton R., Del Vecchio C, Zupin L, Crovella S., Unraveling the Role of Sex Hormones on Keratinocyte Functions in Human Inflammatory Skin Diseases. Int J Mol Sci. 2022 Mar 15; 23(6): 3132.[4]

fibroblasts that produce collagen and hyaluronic acid. One cool fact about hyaluronic acid is that it can bind over 1,000 times its weight in water, which is why it's such a fantastic product for boosting skin hydration.

Sebaceous glands in the dermis produce an oily substance called sebum, and, like many other parts of the skin, have receptors which are influenced by sex hormones. Starting around puberty, sebaceous glands increase in size, and begin to secrete sebum, with the most sebum secreted between 15 and 35 years of age.[5] While sebum acts to keep the skin moisturized, excess amounts can cause the skin to become oily and lead to breakouts.

The subcutaneous layer

The subcutaneous layer, or superficial fascia, is the deepest layer of skin, made of connective tissue and adipose (fat) tissue. It functions as energy storage and provides insulation and cushioning. It also contains skin appendages like hair follicles, sensory neurons and blood vessels.

How hormones affect our skin

Oestrogen

Oestrogen has multiple roles in the skin and is involved in collagen formation, skin hydration (through hyaluronic acid production), wound healing and skin thickness – it is essentially an anti-ageing hormone.[6] It also plays a part in hair growth, influencing the hair follicle life cycle – many women notice they have thicker, better-looking hair during pregnancy, thanks to oestrogen.[7] One downside is that it also regulates pigmentation in the skin, and high levels of oestrogen, for example around ovulation and during pregnancy, can cause patches of skin to become darker than the surrounding skin, known as hyperpigmentation.[8]

Progesterone

The role of progesterone in skin and hair is less clear, but also plays a role in the prevention of skin ageing by reducing the breakdown of collagen, helping to keep skin firm and encouraging the production of new skin cells (keratinocytes), supporting the skin renewal process.[9] Progesterone also increases sebum production, which could potentially trigger breakouts.[10]

Androgens

Androgens, often referred to as 'male hormones', such as testosterone, also influence the skin. Across the menstrual cycle the release of testosterone stays fairly low and steady, with a small peak around ovulation. Androgens, of all the hormones, have the biggest impact on sebum production – and increased levels can lead to noticeably oilier skin, which may progress to acne when combined with dead skin cells and overgrowth of bacteria.

In some women, high levels of testosterone cause growth of coarse and dark hair in certain parts of the body, such as the chin, neck and chest, as well as hair loss from the scalp. This is the case for many women with PCOS, who can experience various hair and skin symptoms, including acne, excessive hair growth (hirsutism) and hair loss (alopecia) as a result of high testosterone. In PCOS, these skin and hair changes are largely driven by raised male hormones (hyperandrogenism) and insulin resistance. So, efforts and interventions to reduce testosterone and improve insulin sensitivity, through nutrition and lifestyle, will likely positively impact skin and hair symptoms. These methods include resistance training,[11] following a high-fibre, low-GI diet,[12] and increasing protein intake.[13] That said, PCOS acne can be pretty stubborn (take it from me!), and for cases of acne not responding to lifestyle changes and topical treatments, there are other prescription-only treatment options available, including more potent topicals, the pill, Spironolactone and Isotretinoin. Speak to your doctor if your acne has become distressing and you've not been able to get a handle on it with topical skincare.

Note: It's also worth pointing out that acne symptoms fluctuating with the menstrual cycle are not always associated with raised androgens or PCOS. For some women, there is a sensitivity of the skin to circulating hormones, rather than an increase in levels of hormones in the blood.

The skin across the menstrual cycle

Not everyone will experience big changes in their skin during their cycle, but for those who do, understanding the changes can allow some anticipatory skincare tweaks tailored to your skin type. It can help for the first few cycles to keep a diary to see if this matches what you experience.

'My skin is awful in the days leading up to my period. The worst flare-up is the week before and then it calms down two days into my cycle. I get spots predominantly on my face and neck, really bad. Outside of this time, I rarely get spots unless I use a product that is too oily, or I eat too much sugar. My hair gets greasier more quickly during my cycle, too!' – **Nadia, 29**

Menstruation

When you're having your period, oestrogen and progesterone levels are low, and so you may notice your skin is dry and sensitive.[14] [15] If so, opt for a more gentle and hydrating skincare routine. You'll also want to give your skin barrier some love by using ceramides, which are lipids that help lock in moisture and protect your skin. Avoid chemical peels and products with strong active ingredients to prevent further irritation.

* Potential skin changes: Dryness and sensitivity
* Ingredients to consider: Hyaluronic acid, glycerin, ceramides, shea butter and other emollients

Late follicular phase and ovulation

Oestrogen rises, peaking just before ovulation, giving skin a dewy glow – often referred to as the 'ovulation glow' . This is because of oestrogen's role in collagen formation and skin hydration.[16] However, some women may notice their skin is a little more oily at this time and experience breakouts – due to a small increase in testosterone around ovulation. Additionally, higher levels of oestrogen can also stimulate pigment production.[17] [18] So, if you are prone to hyperpigmentation, it is super important to step up the SPF and perhaps include skincare products with ingredients that target pigmentation, such as vitamin C. Oral contraceptives can also cause hyperpigmentation in some women.[19]

* Potential skin changes: Hydration, pigmentation
* Ingredients to consider: High-SPF sunscreen and ingredients that target hyperpigmentation such as vitamin C and niacinamide, liquorice extract and kojic acid

Luteal phase

Progesterone rises and peaks in the luteal phase and typically leads to increased sebum production.[20] Androgens such as testosterone also increase sebum production. While this acts as a protective moisturizer for the skin, excess sebum can combine with dirt and dead skin cells and get trapped in pores – making the perfect place for acne-causing bacteria (*cutibacterium acnes*) to thrive. Levels of androgens rise during puberty in males and females, which is why acne is quite common in this age group – but many adults get it too. Most women report flare-ups of their acne symptoms in the days leading up to, and during, the period – typically around the jawline and chin area.[21] For this reason, hormonal treatment (such as the oral contraceptive pill) may be prescribed to help treat acne in women. If you are noticing acne flares around this time, you could include some preventative acne skincare, with products including ingredients such as salicylic acid, benzoyl peroxide, or a retinol. Balance excess oil by double cleansing with a gel-based or foaming cleanser (although I generally recommend double cleansing all month long!).

* Potential skin changes: Oiliness and breakouts
* Ingredients to consider: Salicylic acid, azelaic acid, benzoyl peroxide, or a retinol (speak to your doctor/

dermatologist about prescription medication and specialist treatments)

ACNE AND NUTRITION

One question I often get asked is if nutrition and diet can improve acne, and the truth is, diet alone is unlikely to cure your acne or prevent breakouts. That said, good nutrition is incredibly important for skin health, but I think it's often easy to assume that our skin issues are a result of something *we* are doing, when in reality skin conditions are hugely complex.

A common concern is that dairy causes acne. There are a few studies that have found a possible link between dairy and acne, but they don't prove a 'cause and effect' link.[22] [23] Interestingly, there may be a higher risk of acne with skimmed milk consumption compared to whole milk.[24] [25] So, while there is a possibility that milk may impact acne risk for some people, this risk seems to be low.

Another common belief is that sugar causes acne. How many times have you heard someone blame a breakout on the chocolate or sweets they enjoyed a few days before? It's not that straightforward, but some observational studies have found that frequently spiking blood glucose levels i.e. a high glycaemic index (or high GI) may increase acne risk due to impact on insulin, insulin-like-growth factor-1 and acne.[26] [27] However the results of these studies have been mixed, and not all have found significant improvements.[28] So, although there may be a potential link between glycaemic index or sugar intake and acne, we certainly don't have enough evidence to say that 'sugar should be avoided'. Nevertheless, here are some simple ways to reduce the glycemic impact of food day-to-day:

* **Where possible, opt for whole foods:** In general, less processed foods have a lower GI, so fill up with veggies, nuts and seeds, whole grains and legumes.

* **Balance your plate:** It's the mix of nutrients that determines the glucose response. Pairing carbs with a protein, extra fibre or healthy fats can help lower the GI of the meal, for example, adding peanut butter and chia seed to your bowl of oatmeal or having smoked salmon and salad with your lunchtime bagel.

* **Focus on fibre:** Choose wholegrain and brown versions of starchy carbs like pasta, rice and bread – the additional fibre will help stabilize blood sugar levels and feed your gut bugs at the same time.

Hair and the menstrual cycle

Just as your skin can change throughout your menstrual cycle, so too can your scalp and hair. As sebum production varies across the menstrual cycle and since sebum and the hair follicle exit from the same opening in the skin, the hair and skin surrounding it may be coated in sebum – making the hair greasy. Research in this area is quite limited (I know, I feel like a broken record), but in general, more women report 'bad hair days' during their period. The interesting thing is, this doesn't seem to be correlated to sebum levels on the scalp or forehead, so there's no clear explanation as to why this would be the case. Of course, as we have discussed in the chapter on body image (page XX), it might be due to a difference in our perception of ourselves and our hair at this time in our cycle.[29]

An indirect way that your menstrual cycle can impact your hair is through iron deficiency anaemia as a result of heavy periods. In fact, for girls and women who menstruate, heavy menstrual bleeding (HMB) is the most common cause of iron deficiency.[30] Common symptoms include tiredness, shortness of breath, heart palpitations, headaches and hair loss.[31] So, if you have very heavy periods and are experiencing any of these symptoms, it's important to get checked out.

Hormonal contraception, hair and skin

You've just read about how hormonal fluctuations during the menstrual cycle can influence our skin and hair, so it makes sense that synthetic hormones in our contraception can as well.

You might have heard that hormonal contraception improves acne and makes your hair look thicker and fuller (or experienced it for yourself). Alternatively, you also may have also heard, or experienced, the opposite – that hormonal contraception worsens acne and leads to hair thinning. It can be confusing, especially when your personal experience is different to that of a friend or what you expected, but the thing is, both scenarios can be true, as different forms of hormonal contraception can improve or worsen skin.

Combined forms of contraception

Forms of contraception containing oestrogen and progesterone, such as the pill, can effectively treat acne and hirsutism.[32] [33] Of course, alongside these beneficial side effects, they come with some negative side effects (see page x) and so using contraception for treating these symptoms specifically is not a first-line therapy.

Progesterone-only contraceptives

Overall, progesterone-only methods, such as implants and the hormonal coil, tend to trigger or worsen acne, hirsutism, alopecia and even rosacea.[34] However, it depends on the type and amount of progestin (the synthetic progesterone used in birth control), as some progestins are more likely to activate androgen receptors and therefore make the skin more oily or lead to excess hair growth, while others do the opposite and block these androgen receptors.[35] Newer progestins, for example norgestimate and desogestrel, are less likely to activate androgen receptors.[36] Whereas hormonal

IUDs with a higher dosage of the progestin levonorgestrel, such as Mirena, can trigger acne in some.[37]

When choosing the best form of hormonal contraception for you, it's important to ask your doctor/healthcare provider about potential side effects and any concerns you may have, including any skin-related worries.

Summary

* The skin is composed of three layers: the epidermis, the dermis and the subcutaneous layer.

* Your skin may change in response to hormonal variations occurring throughout your cycle.

* Breakouts and flare-ups of acne are more common in the premenstrual phase.

* Skin changes, like acne, can be a sign of an underlying hormonal imbalance such as PCOS.

* Sugar doesn't cause or cure acne, but a low-glycemic (low-GI) diet may lead to fewer breakouts and flare-ups of acne.

* The menstrual cycle can impact hair directly, through sebum production and our perception of ourselves, and indirectly, due to hair loss caused by iron deficiency anaemia.

* Different forms of hormonal contraception may improve or worsen skin and hair.

Part 3

Getting Support

We've explored common period problems and red flags to look out for when it comes to your menstrual cycle that might prompt you to seek support from a health professional.

As a refresher, this includes:

* Very heavy bleeding, including passing large clots and flooding
* Bleeding between periods, or after sex
* Irregular or absent periods
* Severe mood changes associated with your menstrual cycle

Essentially, any menstrual cycle symptoms that cause severe disruption to your daily life and stop you from going to work/ school, exercising or socializing should prompt a discussion with a healthcare professional. Everyone's experience with their own menstrual cycle is unique, and when it comes to things like heavy or painful periods, what might not bother one person could be hugely debilitating to another – so, if it's bothering you, get it checked out.

That said, sometimes it can be easier said than done, and I appreciate that many women have not received the support they need from their healthcare providers and oftentimes menstrual cycle-related issues are not taken seriously or passed off as something we should just get on with.

While many GPs and doctors are hugely supportive, we learned from the Women's Health Strategy for England how women have not been listened to when it comes to their pain – being told that heavy and painful periods are 'normal' or that they would 'grow out of them'.[1] Many shared stories of how they spoke to doctors on multiple occasions over many months or years before receiving a diagnosis for conditions such as endometriosis.[2]

It's so important that we are able to discuss any distressing symptoms with our doctors – and that we feel listened to. In our survey, we found that women who are comfortable accessing support from healthcare providers experience less severe menstrual symptoms and feel more supported compared to those who do not feel comfortable engaging with healthcare providers about their menstrual health.[3]

If you are experiencing period problems, the first port of call in the UK will be your GP. At the time of writing, I'm aware that getting time with a GP is easier said than done, but it is worth persisting, as they really can help. From there, if required, you can be referred to an NHS gynaecologist. You can also see gynaecologists through private healthcare. If your problem is urgent, such as very heavy bleeding that is causing you to be unwell, dizzy or sick, then you should go to A&E.

Speaking to your doctor about your menstrual cycle

While it's unfortunate that women often need to advocate for themselves in the doctor's office, and it's absolutely not your responsibility to fix a flawed system, you can take proactive steps to improve your experience and access to healthcare.

Here are some self-advocacy tips to help you make the most of your medical appointments:

1. Keep a symptom diary for at least 2–3 menstrual cycles and bring it with you to the appointment.
2. If you have a number of concerns, talk about the most important thing first, as GPs often have a limited time to spend on each patient.
3. Avoid downplaying the severity of your symptoms, and be sure to tell your healthcare provider how these symptoms are affecting your life.
4. If you are concerned that you have a specific condition (e.g., endometriosis or PCOS), share that concern so that your doctor can address it.
5. If it's possible, request a GP you know and feel comfortable with. If you feel like your health concerns are not being taken seriously, you can ask to see another doctor.
6. If you feel more comfortable, you can bring someone with you to your consultation. Sometimes having some-one with us who we trust can help us feel more confident speaking up.

7. Come prepared with questions you would like to ask – for example, if you will need any tests or investigations, or simply what happens next. However, depending on your symptoms, your doctor may not need to do any specific tests, and if this is the case, you can ask them to explain why.

DO I NEED A HORMONE M.O.T.?

At-home hormone testing kits are becoming increasingly popular, partly due to a rise in at-home testing and Zoom consultations due to the COVID-19 pandemic and long waiting lists. While these tests typically can be a convenient first step to further conversations with your doctor, they do come with their own set of pros and cons.[4]

PROS:

* **Convenience:** You can collect samples in the comfort of your home, avoiding the need for clinic visits, therefore saving time.

* **Early detection:** In some cases these tests can identify potential reproductive issues early, allowing for timely intervention and treatment. This is especially important for those considering delaying parenthood.

* **Informed family planning:** For example, understanding your ovarian reserve with anti-Müllerian hormone (AMH) testing can help you make informed decisions about family planning and fertility treatments, if needed.

* **Guiding fertility treatments:** Test results can help tailor fertility treatment protocols by indicating how your body might respond to certain medications or procedures.

* **Can assist with diagnosis of certain conditions:** While these tests typically cannot diagnose an individual with a

hormone-related condition, the results, in combination with other information – such as symptoms, medical history, and other tests – can be used by a medical professional. They can also be used for monitoring purposes in response to different management strategies.

CONS:

* **Stress and anxiety:** Test results can cause stress and anxiety, especially if they don't meet your expectations.

* **Cost:** Testing can be expensive, particularly through clinics, though home-testing kits can make it more accessible at a lower cost. However, positive or concerning results typically require follow-up testing and consultation with a healthcare provider, which can add additional steps and costs.

* **Uncertain predictions**: Hormone levels and ovarian reserve tests provide estimates, but are not definitive predictors of natural conception. Women with a low ovarian reserve might still conceive naturally, while those with a good reserve can still face fertility issues.

* **False assurance:** 'Normal' results can lead to a false sense of security, potentially delaying the seeking of fertility assistance if other issues are present.

* **Testing variability:** Hormone levels can fluctuate, and interpretations of ovarian reserve tests can vary, leading to inconsistent or ambiguous results.

* **Lack of professional guidance:** While most testing companies offer a doctors report or consultation, not all of them are that comprehensive. Without a healthcare provider's interpretation, it can be challenging to understand the results and their implications fully.

If you are concerned that you have a hormone-related issue, I would first speak to your doctor, who can best support you and guide you through any investigations that you may need. If you're considering doing an at-home test to check if your hormones are balanced, I wouldn't. Your hormones are constantly in flux and, technically, you can't 'balance' them. However, if hormone levels are too high or are too low, that can indicate actual hormone-related conditions, which can't be diagnosed or treated exclusively at home.

Supporting a loved one across the menstrual cycle

Communication is key in any healthy relationship, and that includes discussions around the menstrual cycle (if one or both of you menstruate).

Our survey revealed that nearly 85 per cent of women experience disruptions in their intimate relationships due to menstrual cycles. However, those who feel comfortable seeking support from their partners reported fewer disruptions. Couples therapy, when compared to one-on-one therapy or a waitlist group, was found to be the most effective in improving relationships and alleviating premenstrual distress.[5] I recognize, however, that these 'partner' conversations almost always focus on a cis-male perspective, and the majority of women who took part in this study were in heterosexual relationships, so more research is undoubtedly needed to understand efficacy in same-sex couples.

It isn't only romantic relationships that can benefit from open discussion about periods and the menstrual cycle. You can find support from talking about it to friends, siblings and parents, too. And the more we discuss what's happening in our bodies through the lens of our menstrual cycle, the more normalized it will be, and the less shame people will feel.

Originally I was going to dedicate this section to advising you on how to speak to your partner, friend or parent about your menstrual cycle, and while that is incredibly important, I think that your partner, friend or parent is likely the person who needs the advice more! Whenever I do public talks on the menstrual cycle, there are always one or two people in the audience who ask how they can support their loved one across their menstrual cycle, so this section is for you – the boyfriends, girlfriends, husbands, wives, dads, mums and mates:

1. **Educate yourself:** The good news is that you're here, reading this book, so that essentially ticks off the first step. I encourage you to dip in and out of each section to learn what happens across a 'typical' menstrual cycle and how that might affect your loved one's energy levels, mood, nutrition, sleep, etc.
2. **Ask questions:** Your loved one's experience of their cycle will be unique and may differ slightly from the examples in this book. Ask and listen to their needs at different points in the cycle, whether it's through understanding, patience or practical support.
3. **Don't assume it's 'just hormones':** Never dismiss how they feel because of their cycle or their hormones. Their mood and emotions may be influenced in part by their cycle, but research tells us that social support may be a stronger influence,[6] so how you support them matters more.
4. **Get involved:** If your loved one (this one is most likely to be your partner!) is comfortable, they can share through a calendar or period-tracking app where they're at in their cycle. This might make it easier for you to support them or plan activities.

Managing periods in the workplace

Until recently, periods (and women's health in general) was rarely discussed in the context of the workplace and, in many cases, was (and still can be) a taboo subject.

However, thankfully, things seem to be changing, and in 2023 the British Standards Institute published a guide on menstruation, menstrual health and menopause in the workplace.[7] The aim of this guide is to help businesses support employees who menstruate, or experience menopausal symptoms, by offering guidance on workplace adjustments, education and awareness, as well as policies that foster inclusivity.

In the same year, Spain introduced paid menstrual leave, providing 3–5 days of menstrual-related absence per month. This policy aligns with similar ones in Japan, Indonesia and Zambia.[8] However, the effectiveness and usage of these policies vary, sparking debate about their impact. On one hand, menstrual leave can reduce stigma by encouraging open discussions, and benefit the health of those who menstruate, including individuals with conditions like endometriosis and PMDD. On the other hand, it may reinforce sexist beliefs and discrimination, perpetuate menstrual stigma – that you have to closet yourself away and avoid others when menstruating – and negatively affect the gender wage gap.[9] At this stage, we should closely observe and learn from countries that have implemented menstrual leave policies, thoroughly assessing their advantages and disadvantages.

Regardless of the specific implementation strategies, the fact of the matter remains the same: no one can perform at their best when in discomfort or when their basic needs aren't met at work, so it is crucial that employers work to create better conditions, policies and resources for their employees who menstruate.

The scale of the problem

In our survey, we found that 91 per cent of people believe that their work is disrupted by their menstrual cycle symptoms, 21 per cent of these describing this disruption as severe or very severe.[10] In the last year, 32 per cent report taking time off work to manage their menstrual symptoms, some up to 5 days, and when they do take time off, 2.5 per cent use annual leave and 3.5 per cent take it as unpaid leave. In addition to absenteeism, the impact of present-eeism (working while sick) in a state of low productivity, such as reduced work volume and working hours due to menstrual symptoms, was reported by 76 per cent of women.[11] From an economic standpoint, menstrual symptoms lead to significant productivity losses, costing around $4,333 per person each year in the US and about ¥491.1 billion annually in Japan.[12] And these figures don't even include those who have had to stop working, turn down promotions, or quit their jobs because of menstrual health issues, so the actual impact is likely even greater.

Menstrual-health adjustments in the workplace

If you work in HR, or wish to submit a proposal to your HR department, here are some steps your organization can take to create more comfortable working experiences and make workplaces more menstruation-friendly:

Education and awareness: One of the best ways an organization can support its employees is by creating an open, supportive environment where talking about periods is encouraged. This begins with senior leaders and managers, including male colleagues, to understand and acknowledge how coworkers can be supported across their menstrual cycle. Additionally, hosting educational sessions and providing information resources for all employees can significantly increase awareness and understanding across the organization.

Flexible working practices and policies: While debate remains regarding the introduction of menstrual leave policies, employers should ensure their existing policies have clear guidance that allows for menstrual-related absence – without penalizing employees or expecting them to take unpaid leave or annual leave days. Allowing people who menstruate to work from home or have flexible working hours may also help reduce absenteeism, and presenteeism, and improve productivity. Allowing breaks or medical appointments during working hours can make it more comfortable for women to work during their period.

Practical considerations: Companies might consider some of these practical measures in the workplace.

- Free period products in the toilets or an 'emergency supplies' cupboard – to help with the logistical (and financial) challenges that come with having a period.
- Ensuring all staff have access to toilets and discrete places to change clothes. Ideally, lockers should be provided to store period products and any spare clothes they may need.
- Consulting staff on uniform design, including consideration of colours that better hide menstrual leaking, looser fitting and/or materials that stretch to better accommodate bloating.*
- Authorizing access to pain-management strategies such as heat pads and painkillers.

---

* I can confirm that NHS scrubs, while looser fitting, are not period proof.

Appendix: Common Conditions That Cause Period Problems

While each of these conditions deserves a full chapter (or book) to themselves, the purpose of this section is to give you a reference point when I discuss various period problems throughout the book.

For information on PMS and PMDD, see Chapter x.

HA is covered Chapter XX.

Polycystic ovary syndrome (PCOS)

Polycystic ovary syndrome (PCOS) is a common hormone condition that affects 10 per cent of women of reproductive age.[1] Because it is a syndrome (a collection of symptoms), this means those with PCOS may all present differently, with their own symptom profile.

Symptoms of PCOS

These vary from person to person. Some women may have several more severe symptoms, whereas others may experience these more mildly.

* Irregular periods or none at all
* Difficulties getting pregnant
* Difficulty lose weight

* Excessive hair growth (hirsutism), often on the top lip, chin, nipples and stomach
* Thinning of hair and hair loss
* Acne or oily skin
* Patches of dark thick skin (*acanthosis nigricans*) in your armpit or around your groin or neck
* Anxiety, depression, mood swings and low self-esteem

What causes PCOS?

The cause of PCOS is unknown. It is likely to be multifactorial, with both genetic and environmental factors playing a part. However, the main drivers are thought to be due to:

* Raised androgen levels: Many women with PCOS have slightly higher than normal levels of testosterone.[2] High levels of testosterone can both cause, and be a symptom, of PCOS and can impact your insulin levels, periods and ovulation.
* Insulin resistance: Insulin resistance is a common feature in many women with PCOS (up to 80 per cent).[3] These higher levels of insulin can interfere with sex hormones, leading to excess testosterone production, which in turn causes anovulation (failure of the ovaries to release an egg) and irregular periods. It also increases the risk of Type 2 diabetes and cardiovascular disease.
* Inflammation: Women with PCOS typically have more markers of inflammation in the body, suggesting that low-grade, chronic inflammation plays a role.[4]

How is PCOS diagnosed?

To be diagnosed with PCOS, a person must have at least 2 of the following 3 conditions:

1. Irregular or absent periods
2. Evidence of excess androgens (or 'male hormones') either on a blood test or signs such as excess body/facial hair and/or acne
3. Presence of multiple follicles or cysts on the ovaries*

Management of PCOS

Lifestyle modification is often recommended as first-line treatment for women with PCOS. This can include:

* **Nutrition:** There is no specific diet you need to follow, but it's advisable to opt for regular, balanced meals. Include protein from sources like meat, fish, eggs, tofu, legumes and nuts to help with weight management and improve glucose levels.[5] [6] Add omega-3 fatty acids from oily fish, chia seeds and flaxseeds to combat inflammation. Enjoy low glycaemic (low-GI) complex carbohydrates like wholegrain bread, oats and grains to slow glucose absorption, stabilize energy levels and manage cravings.
* **Supplementation:** Inositol is a popular and effective supplement which can help with regulating testosterone production, lowering high blood pressure and blood lipid levels, and improving egg quality and chances of conception in women with PCOS. Studies suggest that the 40:1 ratio of myo- to d-chiro-inositol is the most beneficial.[7] Other supplements you may want to consider if you have PCOS

---

* Despite the name, having polycystic ovaries on an ultrasound does not necessarily mean that you have PCOS (without the other symptoms). Polycystic ovaries are also not necessary to diagnose the syndrome. As such, lots of people believe the name should be changed. (Azziz R. Polycystic Ovary Syndrome: What's in a Name? *The Journal of Clinical Endocrinology & Metabolism*. 2014 Apr 1;99(4):1142–5.)

include vitamin D, omega 3, magnesium and folic acid (if you're planning to conceive). Before taking any supplements, remember to speak to your doctor, a registered dietitian or a registered nutritionist to ensure it's safe to do so.

* **Weight management:** In some cases, weight loss is advisable for women with PCOS who are overweight or have obesity, and this can be effective for managing symptoms. However, those with PCOS may experience weight gain/difficulty losing weight due to insulin resistance and cravings, changes to metabolism, dysregulated hunger hormones and disordered eating.[8] [9]

* **Physical activity:** Regular physical activity may improve ovulation, menstrual cycle regularity, weight management and insulin resistance in women with PCOS.[10] [11]

* **Prioritizing stress management:** People with PCOS are more sensitive to the impact of stress, and research suggests they tend to have higher levels of the stress hormone cortisol than people without PCOS.[12] [13] Try to include stress management strategies in your daily routine, such as meditation, mindfulness practices and guided breathing exercises.

* **Optimizing sleep:** Sleep disturbances are more common in women with PCOS than those without,[14] and lack of sleep can have negative effects on symptoms of PCOS, so make sure to optimize sleep where possible.

Medical management of PCOS

Depending on your symptoms, you may be offered medication such as metformin (a insulin-sensitizing drug) or hormonal contraceptives. Oftentimes women are recommended the pill, and I think there is a perception (judging from social media) that this is given as a 'quick fix' or to cover up symptoms, when that isn't the case. The pill does not 'reset' your period or your hormones, but it can be helpful in some cases of PCOS to keep the womb lining thin (and reduce the risk of endometrial hyperplasia* and cancer) and help with certain symptoms such as excess hair growth and acne.[15] [16] Other hormonal options are available. Some women may also wish to have some assistance with fertility and there are options for that also.

Endometriosis

Endometriosis is a condition where cells similar to the ones in the lining of the womb grow elsewhere in the body, most commonly within the pelvis, but it can also affect other areas of the body. These cells respond to hormone fluctuations that occur across the menstrual cycle, which can cause pain and inflammation in the surrounding tissue. Globally, it is thought to affect 10 per cent (190 million) girls and women of reproductive age.[17]

Symptoms of endometriosis

The most common symptoms include:

* Very painful periods
* Pain in your tummy or pelvis, normally worse around your period
* Heavy periods
* Pain during or after sex
* Pain on opening your bowels or going for a wee (or blood in urine/stool)

---

* Endometrial hyperplasia is a condition where the lining of the womb (endometrium) becomes abnormally thickened. This is not cancer, but in some cases can lead to cancer of the lining of the womb (endometrial cancer).

* Difficulty getting pregnant
* Fatigue

What causes endometriosis?

There are several theories about the cause of endometriosis. It is possible that a combination of the following factors could be at play in some of those affected by the condition:

* **Retrograde menstruation:** Menstrual blood, and endometrial cells, flow backwards into the pelvis instead of leaving the body, causing cells to implant on pelvic organs.
* **Lymphatic or circulatory spread:** Endometrial tissue might travel to distant parts of the body, like the lungs or brain, through the lymphatic system or bloodstream.
* **Genetics:** Some people may be more likely to develop endometriosis because of their genes.
* **Cell change (metaplasia):** Cells in the pelvic area change into cells similar to those lining the uterus.
* **Environment:** Toxins in the environment might impact the body and immune system, leading to endometriosis.
* **Immune dysfunction:** Women with endometriosis may have reduced immunity.

How is endometriosis diagnosed?

The only definitive way to diagnose endometriosis is via laparoscopic, or keyhole, surgery to see inside the pelvic cavity. As this is quite invasive, it is one of the reasons why there is usually such a delay from onset of symptoms to diagnosis. There is ongoing research into less invasive ways of testing. Sometimes, endometriosis can be seen on high-quality ultrasound depending on where it is (e.g., ovarian endometriosis) and if done by healthcare professionals trained to look for and see endometriosis. A negative scan does not rule out endometriosis.

Management of endometriosis

There is no cure for endometriosis, but early diagnosis and treatment can slow or stop the disease from getting worse and reduce long-term pain and discomfort. Treatment is also individual, depending on the nature and severity of symptoms and wishes for future conception.

Non-hormonal treatments:

* **Heat therapy** (such as warm baths or heating pads)
* **TENS machines** (as discussed on page XX).
* **Painkillers:** Anti-inflammatory painkillers such as ibuprofen and mefenamic acid may be better than paracetamol. Codeine is an alternative. However, not everyone can take these medications. Some hospitals and trusts have specialized pain clinics providing advice and support to people in chronic pain.
* **Tranexamic acid:** This can be helpful in reducing heavy periods.
* **Physiotherapy:** Physiotherapists can develop a programme of exercise and relaxation techniques designed to help strengthen pelvic floor muscles, reduce pain, and manage stress and anxiety.
* **Psychological support:** Psychologists and counsellors can play an important role by helping those with endometriosis cope with the feelings of confusion, chronic pain, fertility problems and frustration that often accompany this disease. If you wish to go down this route, speak to your GP, who should be able to refer you to a counselling service.

✳ Nutritional support

- **A Mediterranean-style diet** has been associated with improved endometriosis-associated pain.[18]
- In particular, **omega-3-rich foods** (such as oily fish) and **antioxidants** (such a vitamins C and E) may help with pain.[19] [20] [21] [22] We need more studies to confirm the use of vitamin E and C supplementation in endometriosis, but a great place to start is looking at your diet. Vitamin E can be found in nuts, seeds, olive oil, salmon and avocados, while citrus fruits, bell peppers, berries and tomatoes all contain high levels of vitamin C.
- **Vitamin D:** Clinical studies have shown that vitamin D supplementation significantly decreases pelvic pain in women with endometriosis.[23] In the UK, it is advisable to take 10mcg per day from October to March.
- **Gut health:** Research suggests that gut bacteria are linked to inflammation, estrogen levels and immune function, which can influence the development and progression of endometriosis.[24] [25] Make gut health a priority by aiming for 30g of fibre per day from a variety of plant-based foods.
- **Gluten:** Despite a lack of good-quality evidence for using a gluten-free diet to improve symptoms of endometriosis, one study did find positive results.[26] Another study noted a slightly increased risk of coeliac disease in those with endometriosis, although the reason for this is not known.[27] If you are concerned or have a family history, get tested.
- **IBS and Low FODMAP:** Between 36 per cent and 52 per cent of people with endometriosis have IBS.[28] [29] [30] Preliminary data suggests that a low FODMAP diet (a therapeutic diet used in IBS) may assist women struggling with bowel symptoms such

as bloating and loose stools in endometriosis.[31] Seek support and guidance from a trained registered dietitian.

Hormonal treatments

Hormone treatments such as the pill, the mini pill, the hormonal coil or synthetic hormones (GnRH analogues) are often used to reduce endometriosis symptoms. If you are offered the choice of hormone treatment, you may want to discuss with your doctor what it involves, the pros and cons, and possible side effects.

Surgical treatments

Surgery can alleviate pain by removing endometriosis, dividing adhesions, or removing cysts. Laparoscopic (or keyhole) surgery is used to investigate and diagnose endometriosis, and in *some* cases, the endometriosis can be treated in the same operation. Unfortunately, even if the endometriosis is excised, it can grow back in the future. More radical surgery can be considered if a woman has not responded to drug treatments or conservative surgery and is not planning to start a family. Radical surgery refers to a hysterectomy or oophorectomy (removal of the ovaries).

Adenomyosis

Adenomyosis is a condition where endometrial tissue, which normally lines the inside of the uterus, grows into the muscular wall of the uterus (myometrium). This tissue behaves similarly to the normal endometrial lining, thickening, breaking down, and bleeding with each menstrual cycle. This abnormal growth can lead to an enlarged uterus and cause symptoms such as heavy menstrual bleeding, severe cramping and chronic pelvic pain. Adenomyosis is similar to endometriosis in that both involve the presence of endometrial-like tissue outside the uterine lining, but in adenomyosis, the tissue is embedded within the uterine muscle. While endometriosis remains insufficiently under-stood and under-researched, even less is known, or done, about adenomyosis.

Symptoms of adenomyosis[32]

* Painful periods
* Heavy periods
* Bleeding between periods
* Pelvic pain
* Bloating
* Pain during sex
* Bladder and bowel symptoms (such as urinary frequency and constipation)*
* Difficulty getting pregnant

Some women with adenomyosis have no symptoms at all.

What causes it adenomyosis?

The exact cause of adenomyosis is unclear, but several factors may contribute to its development. One theory is that the invasive tissue growth is possibly triggered by uterine inflammation related to childbirth or other trauma (adenomyosis is more common if you have had a baby). Another possibility is that adenomyosis could develop from embryonic stem cells in the uterus that differentiate improperly, leading to the presence of endometrial tissue in the muscle wall.[33]

---

* These symptoms are caused by pressure on the bladder and bowel due to having an enlarged uterus

How is adenomyosis diagnosed?

Adenomyosis can be diagnosed on transvaginal ultrasound scan or MRI scan.[34] Focal adenomyosis (known as adenomyomas) are sometimes mistaken as fibroids (see page XX).

Management of adenomyosis

Less research and fewer clinical trials have been done on adenomyosis and effective treatment options. However, treatment options include:

Non-hormonal

* **Heat therapy** (such as warm baths or heating pads)
* **TENS machines** (as discussed on page XX)
* **Painkillers:** NSAIDs and paracetamol are often used to help ease painful periods and pelvic pain related to this condition. Mefenamic acid may be prescribed to reduce both pain and bleeding.
* Tranexamic acid: This can be helpful in reducing heavy periods.
* **Nutrition:** Overall, there is a significant lack of research about nutrition and adenomyosis to date, but applying many of the principles that we know about endometriosis can be helpful, such as including anti-inflammatory foods – think colourful fruits and veggies, nuts and seeds, olive oil, oily fish, herbs and spices!

Hormonal

Various hormonal therapies are available which, include the combined oral contraceptive pill (COCP) and progesterone-only pill (POP), the hormonal coil, and GnRH analogues. The Mirena coil is generally considered to be the best primary therapy due to overall success rates and low side effects compared to other treatments.[35]

Surgical

* Uterine artery embolization (a minimally invasive, interventional radiological technique which works by reducing blood flow and the size of the uterus)
* Hysterectomy (removal of the uterus)
* For more focal collections of adenomyosis, there may also be other surgical options

Fibroids

A fibroid is a non-cancerous (benign) growth of the womb (uterus). They are also called uterine myomas or leiomyomas. Their size can vary, and you can have just one fibroid or multiple fibroids at the same time.

There are different types of fibroids:

* **Intramural fibroids** – the most common type of fibroid, which develop in the muscle wall of the uterus
* **Subserosal fibroids** – thee develop outside the wall of the uterus into the pelvis and can become very large
* **Submucosal fibroids** – these develop in the muscle layer beneath the uterus's inner lining and grow into the cavity of the uterus
* In some cases, subserosal or submucosal fibroids are attached to the womb with a narrow stalk of tissue. These are known as **pedunculated fibroids**.[36]

Black women are diagnosed with fibroids about 3 times more

often than white women. They also tend to develop fibroids earlier, have larger and more numerous fibroids, and experience more severe symptoms.[37]

Symptoms of fibroids

Fibroids cause no symptoms in 50 per cent of women.[38]
Women who do have symptoms may experience:

* Heavy periods
* Painful periods
* Pelvic pain
* Lower back pain
* Pressure symptoms such as a frequent need to urinate and constipation
* Pain or discomfort during sex
* Fertility problems
* In some cases, a noticeable enlargement of the lower abdomen

What causes fibroids?

The exact cause of fibroids is unknown, but researchers believe multiple factors may contribute, including hormonal (oestrogen and progesterone) and genetic factors (family history). Fibroids grow rapidly during pregnancy when hormone levels are high and shrink with anti-hormone medication or after menopause when hormone levels drop.

How are fibroids diagnosed?

If your doctor suspects fibroids, they'll usually carry out a pelvic examination to look for any obvious signs. Ultrasound is typically used to diagnose fibroids, and in some cases MRI when more detailed information is required. Hysteroscopy, where a small, lighted telescope is inserted through the cervix into the uterus, may be used. This allows your doctor to look inside your womb and take tissue samples (biopsies), if needed.

Management of fibroids

Treatment depends on the symptoms, size and location of the fibroids, your age, and any future pregnancy plans. If your fibroids are not causing any symptoms, they do not usually require treatment.

Lifestyle

* While diet won't 'cure' fibroids, some research has linked the increased consumption of fruit, vegetables and dairy products with a lower risk of developing fibroids.[39] [40] Low vitamin D levels and alcohol consumption may also increase the risk.[41] [42] [43] [44]
* Fibroids can cause heavy menstrual bleeding, which can lead to low iron levels and to anaemia. This can be checked easily on a blood test, but stores can also be topped up through diet and supplements.

Medical

* **Tranexamic acid**: This can help reduce bleeding.
* **Anti-inflammatory medicines**: Ibuprofen and mefenamic acid ease period pain and reduce prostaglandin levels, which contribute to heavy and painful periods.
* **Combined oral contraceptive pill (COCP)**: This can help you to have lighter periods and reduces period pain.
* **Hormonal coil (IUS) e.g., Mirena**: This by making the womb lining thinner and reducing bleeding.

* **Progestogen tablets/injections:** You can take progestogen tablets at certain times in your cycle or have the progestogen-only injection. The injection, usually used for contraception, tends to reduce or stop periods.
* **GnRH analogues:** These lower oestrogen levels, thereby shrinking fibroids, but can cause menopausal symptoms and increase the risk of osteoporosis. They should only used in the short term, therefore – for example, to reduce the size of fibroids before surgery.[45]

Surgical

Surgery to remove your fibroids may be considered if your symptoms are particularly severe and medicine has been ineffective. The main surgical and non-surgical procedures are:

* **Myomectomy:** Surgical removal of fibroids, preserving the uterus and fertility.
* **Hysterectomy:** Removal of the uterus.
* **Endometrial ablation:** Destroys the lining of the uterus to reduce heavy menstrual bleeding, but is not effective for large fibroids.[46]
* **Uterine artery embolization:** Small particles are injected into the arteries supplying the uterus, cutting off blood flow to fibroids and causing them to shrink.[47] [48]

Other, alternative procedures may be offered.

Polyps

Polyps are common growths that extend from delicate tissues, often appearing stalk-like or elongated and fragile. They can develop in various body parts, including the large intestine, nasal passages, uterus (endometrial or uterine polyps) and cervix (cervical polyps). They are considered benign, but a very small percentage may be pre-cancerous or cancerous.[49][50]

Symptoms of polyps

It's common not to have any symptoms of polyps, and they are often discovered incidentally during a smear test or ultrasound scan. However, polyps can cause symptoms such as:

* Bleeding between periods
* Bleeding after sex
* Bleeding after the menopause
* Heavy periods

What causes polyps?

The exact cause is unknown, but may be linked to increased levels of oestrogen and chronic inflammation.

How are polyps diagnosed?

Cervical polyps can be seen upon examination of the cervix. Endometrial polyps can be diagnosed on an ultrasound scan, but other scans may be required, such as sonohysterography (an ultrasound scan where fluid is inserted into the uterus to give a better view of the lining of the womb).

Management of polyps

If polyps are not causing symptoms, it's often enough to monitor them to see if they grow in size or begin to cause symptoms. Your gynaecologist will help you make the decision that is right for you. Removing cervical polyps is usually a simple procedure that a doctor can perform in their office. Endometrial polyps are removed by hysteroscopy. Once removed, endometrial and/or cervical polyps may recur. It is possible that you might need to undergo further treatments in the future, although this is not usually the case.

Hypothalamic amenorrhoea (HA)

Hypothalamic amenorrhoea (HA), also called functional hypothalamic amenorrhoea (FHA), is thought to be responsible for 20–35 per cent of cases of secondary amenorrhoea (i.e., when someone has previously had a period, but now it's gone vs never having had a period), with rates higher in athletic women.[51]

Symptoms of hypothalamic amenorrhoea

* Irregular or no period(s)
* Very light periods
* Low sex drive
* Feeling cold often
* Low mood
* Difficulty sleeping
* Increased hunger
* Low energy

Unfortunately, the consequences of not having a period can lead to serious consequences if not addressed. Key risks associated with HA include:

* Increased cardiovascular disease (CVD) risk due to low oestrogen levels[52]

* Decreased bone density, increasing the risk of osteoporosis or osteopenia, and fractures[53]
* Higher levels of depression and anxiety[54]
* Difficulty getting pregnant[55]

What causes hypothalamic amenorrhoea?

The simplest explanation for HA is that the body lacks enough energy and is experiencing excessive stress. As a result, it conserves energy by shutting down the reproductive system. HA can be brought about through restrictive dieting, excessive exercise, weight loss, stress, or a combination of these factors. Mutations have been found in a number of proteins involved in the regulation of the menstrual cycle in women with HA, suggesting a potential genetic susceptibility.[56]

How is hypothalamic amenorrhoea diagnosed?

HA is a diagnosis of exclusion, which means that all other medical conditions that could potentially cause loss of periods must be ruled out first. Diagnostic tests to do this may be a physical exam, ultrasound, pregnancy test, blood tests and occasionally a CT or MRI to check the brain. Blood tests may come back normal in HA, but oftentimes oestrogen is low and LH and FSH levels will be low, or on the lower end of normal.[57] Other hormones may also be downregulated.

The process may be long and difficult, but getting the right diagnosis is key in finding the most appropriate treatment options for you. For example, HA is often misdiagnosed as PCOS, and while having both conditions is also possible, mislabelling women with PCOS prevents them from receiving care for their actual issue – and, as we have seen, HA left untreated can lead to multiple health consequences.

Note: This condition can be difficult to detect, especially if using hormonal contraception that masks natural menstrual cycles.

Management of hypothalamic amenorrhoea

Addressing the root cause of HA is ultimately the only way we can restore periods. This involves:

* **Nutrition:** For HA, this means increasing daily calorie intake and ensuring adequate consumption of protein, carbohydrates and fats. It is not just what or how much we eat that is important in the context of HA, but also *when* we eat, so aim to avoid long periods without eating (see page XX). If weight loss has occurred, restoring weight or gaining weight may be necessary, although HA can affect women of all body shapes and sizes.
* **Exercise:** While some approaches suggest cutting out exercise completely (and this may be suitable for some people), consider at least reducing the volume and intensity of exercise, avoid fasted training, and take full rest days.
* **Sleep and stress:** Those with HA should try to optimize sleep (see page XXX) and aim to reduce as much external stress as much as possible.

Beyond lifestyle modifications, occasionally medical treatment such as hormone replacement therapy may be advised.

When it comes to HA, the good news is that it can be reversed. However, it can be a long and frustrating process, and one that is best undertaken with the guidance of a registered dietitian or registered nutritionist with expertise in HA. Medical and psychological input may also be required.

Further reading and resources

Condition-specific

Endometriosis

The Endometriosis Foundation

www.theendometriosisfoundation.org

Endometriosis UK

www.endometriosis-uk.org

Support networks for those affected by endometriosis, providing the support and information they need to understand the condition and take control.

PCOS

Verity

www.verity-pcos.org.uk

A charity that helps support women with PCOS from pre-diagnosis through to an understanding of long-term health risks.

PMS and PMDD

International Association for Premenstrual Disorders (IAPMD)

www.iapmd.org

Support, information, and resources for women and AFAB individuals with premenstrual dysphoric disorder (PMDD) and premenstrual exacerbation (PME).

Mind

www.mind.org.uk

Supportive and reliable information to help you with mental health concerns.

Adenomyosis

Adenomyosis Support UK (Facebook group)

Adenomyosis support for UK sufferers.

Fibroids

British Fibroid Trust

www.britishfibroidtrust.org.uk

A UK-based voluntary not-for-profit patient support group which is run by volunteers, who provide balanced information, independent of healthcare providers' interests.

POI (premature ovarian insufficiency)

The Daisy Network

www.daisynetwork.org

The Daisy Network is dedicated to providing information and support to women diagnosed with premature ovarian insufficiency.

Contraception

Contraception Choices

www.contraceptionchoices.org

The Low Down

www.thelowdown.com

Books

The Female Factor by Dr Hazel Wallace

Dealing with Period Problems by Dr Anita Mitra

Blood: The Science, Medicine and Mythology of Menstruation by Dr Jen Gunter

No Period. Now What?: A Guide to Regaining Your Cycles and Improving Your Fertility by Nicola J. Rinaldi, Stephanie G. Buckler and Lisa Sanfilippo Waddell

Australia

Condition-specific

Endometriosis

Endometriosis Australia

www.endometriosisaustralia.org

Endometriosis Australia is a nationally accredited charity that raises awareness, educates and funds research for endometriosis.

QENDO

www.qendo.org.au

Established in 1988, QENDO advocates for those affected by endometriosis and other pelvic health related conditions across Australia and New Zealand. QENDO is a peak organization for those affected by endometriosis, adenomyosis, PCOS, infertility or pelvic pain, by lobbying for national programs, better healthcare access, support, offering them the tools, services and programs to understand and take control of their health.

PCOS

Jean Hailes for Women's Health

www.jeanhailes.org.au

Jean Hailes for Women's Health is a national not-for-profit organization dedicated to improving women's health across Australia through every life stage.

PMS and PMDD

International Association for Premenstrual Disorders (IAPMD)

www.iapmd.org

Support, information, and resources for women and AFAB individuals with premenstrual dysphoric disorder (PMDD) and premenstrual exacerbation (PME).

Adenomyosis

QUENDO

QENDO is a peak organization for those affected by endometriosis, adenomyosis, PCOS, infertility or pelvic pain

Adenomyosis Australia

www.adenomyosis.org.au

An organization that gives women with adenomyosis a voice as well as a helping hand so they may combat this condition and receive assistance along the way.

POI (premature ovarian insufficiency)

The Daisy Network

www.daisynetwork.org

The Daisy Network is dedicated to providing information and support to women diagnosed with premature ovarian insufficiency.

South Africa

Endometriosis

Endometriosis South Africa (Facebook group)

A safe space where women guide each other through the struggles of endometriosis.

PCOS

PCOS Support Group South Africa (Facebook group)

This is a group for South African Women suffering with PCOS, endometriosis, infertility, where they can get support from fellow sisters.

PMS and PMDD

International Association for Premenstrual Disorders (IAPMD)

www.iapmd.org

Support, information and resources for women and AFAB individuals with premenstrual dysphoric disorder (PMDD) and premenstrual exacerbation (PME).

Fibroids

The White Dress Project

www.thewhitedressproject.org

To galvanize support and promote national awareness about the fibroid epidemic among people domestically and globally through education, research, and advocacy.

POI (premature ovarian insufficiency)

The Daisy Network

www.daisynetwork.org

The Daisy Network is dedicated to providing information and support to women diagnosed with premature ovarian insufficiency.

India

Endometriosis

Indian Centre for Endometriosis

www.endometriosis-india.com

An educational resource about endometriosis, for patients as well as physicians.

PCOS

The PCOS Society of India

www.pcosindia.org

PMS and PMDD

International Association for Premenstrual Disorders (IAPMD)

www.iapmd.org

Support, information, and resources for women and AFAB individuals with premenstrual dysphoric disorder (PMDD) and premenstrual exacerbation (PME).

Fibroids

The Fibroid Foundation

www.fibroidfoundation.org

The Fibroid Foundation is the premier fibroids nonprofit, supporting and amplifying the voice of those with uterine fibroids.

The White Dress Project

www.thewhitedressproject.org

To galvanize support and promote national awareness about the fibroid epidemic among people domestically and globally through education, research, and advocacy.

POI (premature ovarian insufficiency)

The Daisy Network

www.daisynetwork.org

The Daisy Network is dedicated to providing information and support to women diagnosed with premature ovarian insufficiency.

US

HealthyWomen

www.healthywomen.org

The nation's leading nonprofit educating and empowering women to make decisions about their health care.

Endometriosis

EndoFound: Endometriosis Foundation of America

www.endofound.org

The Endometriosis Foundation of America strives to provide relevant and cutting-edge information on endometriosis to support those who may be struggling with the disease.

PCOS

PCOS Challenge: The National Polycystic Ovary Syndrome Association

www.pcoschallenge.org

The leading nonprofit support and advocacy organization advancing the cause for people impacted by polycystic ovary syndrome.

PMS and PMDD

International Association for Premenstrual Disorders (IAPMD)

www.iapmd.org

Support, information, and resources for women and AFAB individuals with premenstrual dysphoric disorder (PMDD) and premenstrual exacerbation (PME).

Adenomyosis

Adenomyosis Advice Association

www.adenomyosisadviceassociation.org

The Adenomyosis Advice Association offers free information, advice, and support to people with adenomyosis worldwide

Fibroids

The Fibroid Foundation

www.fibroidfoundation.org

The Fibroid Foundation is the premier fibroids nonprofit, supporting and amplifying the voice of those with uterine fibroids.

POI (premature ovarian insufficiency)

The Daisy Network

www.daisynetwork.org

The Daisy Network is dedicated to providing information and support to women diagnosed with Premature Ovarian Insufficiency

Glossary

Adenomyosis

A condition where the lining of the womb (uterus) starts growing into the muscle in the wall of the womb.

Alopecia

Hair loss that can affect just your scalp or your entire body; can be temporary or permanent.

Amenorrhoea

The absence of menstruation.

Anaemia

A condition in which the blood has a reduced ability to carry oxygen. Iron deficiency anaemia is often caused by heavy menstrual bleeding.

Androgens

Male hormones, like testosterone, that primarily help to regulate sex characteristics in the body; found in both males and females.

Anovulation

Occurs when the ovaries do not release an egg during a menstrual cycle.

Cervical ectropion

When cells from inside the cervical canal move to the outside of the cervix (neck of the womb).

Corpus luteum

A temporary structure that forms on the surface of the ovary after it releases an egg (ovulation).

Dysfunctional uterine bleeding (DUB)

Heavy menstrual bleeding without any obvious structural or systemic pathology.

Dysmenorrhoea

The medical term for painful periods.

Endometrial hyperplasia

A condition where the lining of the womb (endometrium) becomes abnormally thickened. This is not cancer, but in some cases can lead to cancer of the lining of the womb (endometrial cancer).

Endometriosis

A condition where tissue that is similar to the lining of the womb is found in other parts of the body, most commonly in the pelvic cavity.

Endometrium

The tissue that lines the womb.

Fibroids

A non-cancerous (benign) growth of the womb (uterus).

Follicular phase

The first phase of the menstrual cycle and includes the maturation of ovarian follicles to prepare one of them for release during ovulation. The follicular phase starts with the first day of your period and ends with ovulation.

Hirsutism

Excessive growth of 'male' pattern hair that appears on the face, back, chest, stomach and thighs in women.

Hypothalamic amenorrhoea

A condition where the menstrual cycle stops due to abnormal signalling between the brain (hypothalamus) and ovaries, often related to low energy availability.

Hysterectomy

Surgical removal of the uterus.

Intermenstrual bleeding

Bleeding between periods.

Insulin resistance

When cells in your muscles, fat and liver don't respond well to insulin and can't easily take up glucose from your blood.

Laparoscopic surgery

A type of keyhole surgery used to diagnose and treat conditions.

Luteal phase

The second half of the menstrual cycle where the lining of the uterus prepares for implantation and pregnancy. The luteal phase begins at ovulation until the start of the next menstrual period.

Menopause

A point in time 12 months after the final menstrual period.

Menorrhagia

Heavy menstrual bleeding.

Menstruation

The monthly shedding of the lining of your uterus, also called a 'period'.

Oligomenorrhea

Irregular periods.

Oophorectomy

Surgical removal of the ovary/ovaries.

Osteopenia

The stage before osteoporosis when a bone density scan shows you have lower bone density than the average for your age, but not low enough to be classed as osteoporosis.

Osteoporosis

A condition characterized by weak and brittle bones, making you more likely to fracture (break) a bone.

Ovulation

The release of an egg from the ovary.

Polyps

Polyps are growths that protrude out of the surface of delicate skin, usually stalk-like or elongated and quite fragile. An endometrial polyp is where the cell overgrowth is located in the lining (endometrium) of the womb (uterus). A cervical polyp is an overgrowth that develops in the cervix and within the canal that connects the uterus to the vagina.

Post-coital bleeding

Bleeding after sex.

Post-menopausal bleeding

Bleeding 12 months after your last period.

Premature ovarian insufficiency (POI)

Temporary or permanent loss of ovarian function before the age of 40.

Premenstrual dysphoric disorder (PMDD)

A cyclical, hormone-based mood disorder with symptoms arising during the premenstrual, or luteal, phase of the menstrual cycle and subsiding within a few days of menstruation.

Premenstrual syndrome (PMS)

A condition characterized by distressing physical, behavioural and psychological symptoms that recur during the luteal phase of the menstrual cycle and that disappear or improve by the end of the period.

Primary amenorrhoea

When periods have not started by age of 13 or 14 (with no other signs of puberty) or by the age of 15 or 16 (with other signs of puberty such as breast development).

Primary dysmenorrhoea

Painful menstrual periods with no underlying condition.

Secondary amenorrhoea

When menstruation has previously occurred but has stopped.

Secondary dysmenorrhoea

Painful menstrual periods caused by an underlying condition such as endometriosis.

Spotting

Light bleeding from the vagina that is noticeable but not substantial enough to soak a pad or liner.

References

Introduction

1 Regional Health–Americas TL. Menstrual health: a neglected public health problem. *Lancet Reg Health Am.* 2022 Nov 11;15:100399.

2 Department of Health and Social Care. Results of the 'Women's Health – Let's talk about it' survey. 2021.

3 The Period Taboo: A Universal Problem | CARE International [Internet]. 2021 [cited 10 October 2024]. Available from: https://www.care-international.org/stories/period-taboo-universal-problem

4 Thakuri DS, Thapa RK, Singh S, Khanal GN, Khatri RB. A harmful religio-cultural practice (Chhaupadi) during menstruation among adolescent girls in Nepal: Prevalence and policies for eradication. *PLoS One.* 2021 Sep 1;16(9):e0256968.

5 The Food Medic. Perceptions of the menstrual cycle and impact on quality of life, employment, and relationships. [Internet]. October 2024. Available from: https://www.thefoodmedic.co.uk/

6 Schoep ME, Adang EMM, Maas JWM, Bie BD, Aarts JWM, Nieboer TE. Productivity loss due to menstruation-related symptoms: a nationwide cross-sectional survey among 32 748 women. *BMJ Open.* 2019 Jun 1;9(6):e026186.

7 Hearn JH, Bryson K, Barsauskaite L, Bullo S. A COM-B and Theoretical Domains Framework Mapping of the Barriers and Facilitators to Effective Communication and Help-Seeking Among People With, or Seeking a Diagnosis Of, Endometriosis. *Journal of Health Communication.* 2024 Mar 3;29(3):174–86.

8 Zhang L, Losin EAR, Ashar YK, Koban L, Wager TD. Gender Biases in Estimation of Others' Pain. *J Pain.* 2021 Sep;22(9):1048–59.

9 Chen EH, Shofer FS, Dean AJ, Hollander JE, Baxt WG, Robey JL, et al. Gender disparity in analgesic treatment of emergency department patients with acute abdominal pain. *Acad Emerg Med.* 2008 May; 15(5):414–8.

10 Hoffmann DE, Tarzian AJ. The girl who cried pain: a bias against women in the treatment of pain. *J Law Med Ethics.* 2001;29(1):13–27.

11 Chen EH, Shofer FS, Dean AJ, Hollander JE, Baxt WG, Robey JL, et al. Gender disparity in analgesic treatment of emergency department patients with acute abdominal pain. *Acad Emerg Med.* 2008 May;15(5):414–8.

12 Public Health England. Survey reveals women experience severe reproductive health issues [Internet]. 2018 [cited 2024 Jul 6]. Available from: https://www.gov.uk/government/news/survey-reveals-women-experi ence-severe-reproductive-health-issues

13 Research Gate. Why do we still not know what causes PMS? [Internet]. 2016 [cited 2024 Jul 6]. Available from: https://www.researchgate.net/ blog/why-do-we-still-not-know-what-causes-pms

14 Wise J. Women's health: specific assessments to become mandatory in medical training. *BMJ.* 2022 Jul 20;378:o1820.

15 Womersley K, Hockham C, Mullins E. The Women's Health Strategy: ambitions need action and accountability. *BMJ.* 2022 Aug 19;378:o2059.

16 NICHD EKSNI of CH and HD. Menstrual Cycles as a Fifth Vital Sign [Internet]. 2021 [cited 2024 Jul 6]. Available from: https://www. nichd.nih.gov/about/org/od/directors_corner/prev_updates/menstrual-cycles

Part 1: Get to Know Your Cycle

Overview of the menstrual cycle

1 Grieger JA, Norman RJ. Menstrual Cycle Length and Patterns in a Global Cohort of Women Using a Mobile Phone App: Retrospective Cohort Study. *J Med Internet Res.* 2020 Jun 24;22(6):e17109.

2 Bull JR, Rowland SP, Scherwitzl EB, Scherwitzl R, Danielsson KG, Harper J. Real-world menstrual cycle characteristics of more than 600,000 menstrual cycles. *npj Digit Med.* 2019 Aug 27;2(1):1–8.

3 Najmabadi S, Schliep KC, Simonsen SE, Porucznik CA, Egger MJ, Stanford JB. Menstrual bleeding, cycle length, and follicular and luteal phase lengths in women without known subfertility: A pooled analysis of three cohorts. *Paediatr Perinat Epidemiol.* 2020 May;34(3):318–27.

4 Salamonsen LA. Menstrual Fluid Factors Mediate Endometrial Repair. *Front Reprod Health.* 2021 Dec 21;3:779979.

5 Wilcox AJ, Dunson D, Baird DD. The timing of the 'fertile window' in the menstrual cycle: day specific estimates from a prospective study. *BMJ.* 2000 Nov 18;321(7271):1259–62.

6 Durai R, Ng PCH. Mittelschmerz mimicking appendicitis. *Br J Hosp Med* (Lond). 2009 Jul;70(7):419.

7 Soumpasis I, Grace B, Johnson S. Real-life insights on menstrual cycles and ovulation using big data. *Hum Reprod Open.* 2020;2020(2):hoaa011.

8 Popat V, Prodanov T, Calis K, Nelson L. The Menstrual Cycle A Biological Marker of General Health in Adolescents. *Annals of the New York Academy of Sciences.* 2008 Jul 1;1135:43–51.

Tracking your cycle

1 Broad A, Biswakarma R, Harper JC. A survey of women's experiences of using period tracker applications: Attitudes, ovulation prediction and how the accuracy of the app in predicting period start dates affects their feelings and behaviours. *Women's Health* (Lond). 2022;18:17455057 221095246.

2 Zwingerman R, Chaikof M, Jones C. A Critical Appraisal of Fertility and Menstrual Tracking Apps for the iPhone. *J Obstet Gynaecol Can.* 2020 May;42(5):583–90.

3 Al-Rshoud F, Qudsi A, Naffa FW, Al Omari B, AlFalah AG. The Use and Efficacy of Mobile Fertility-tracking Applications as a Method of Contraception: a Survey. *Curr Obstet Gynecol Rep.* 2021;10(2):25–9.

What's normal, what's not

1 NICE Guideline. Menorrhagia | CKS | NICE [Internet]. 2024 [cited 2024 Dec 2]. Available from: https://cks.nice.org.uk/topics/menorr hagia-heavy-menstrual-bleeding/background-information/definition/

2 Quinn SD, Higham J. Outcome Measures for Heavy Menstrual Bleeding. *Women's Health* (Lond). 2016 Jan;12(1):21–6.

3 Menorrhagia (heavy menstrual bleeding) | Health topics A to Z | CKS | NICE [Internet]. [cited 2024 Jul 2]. Available from: https://cks.nice.org.uk/topics/menorrhagia-heavy-menstrual-bleeding/

4 Wear White Again [Internet]. [cited 2024 Oct 10]. Talking Heavy Periods! Available from: https://www.wearwhiteagain.co.uk/hmb-the-lived-experience/

5 Chen CX, Shieh C, Draucker CB, Carpenter JS. Reasons women do not seek health care for dysmenorrhea. *J Clin Nurs.* 2018 Jan;27(1–2):e301–8.

6 Chen CX, Shieh C, Draucker CB, Carpenter JS. Reasons women do not seek health care for dysmenorrhea. *J Clin Nurs.* 2018 Jan;27(1–2):e301–8.

7 Iacovides S, Avidon I, Baker FC. What we know about primary dysmenorrhea today: a critical review. *Hum Reprod Update.* 2015;21(6):762–78.

8 Chen CX, Shieh C, Draucker CB, Carpenter JS. Reasons women do not seek health care for dysmenorrhea. *J Clin Nurs.* 2018 Jan;27(1–2):e301–8.

9 https://drjengunter.com/2018/03/02/comparing-period-cramps-with-heart-attacks-isnt-useful-or-accurate/

10 Iacovides S, Avidon I, Baker FC. What we know about primary dysmenorrhea today: a critical review. *Hum Reprod Update.* 2015;21(6):762–78.

11 Itani R, Soubra L, Karout S, Rahme D, Karout L, Khojah HMJ. Primary Dysmenorrhea: Pathophysiology, Diagnosis, and Treatment Updates. *Korean J Fam Med.* 2022 Mar;43(2):101–8.

12 Marjoribanks J, Ayeleke RO, Farquhar C, Proctor M. Nonsteroidal anti-inflammatory drugs for dysmenorrhoea – Marjoribanks, J – 2015 | Cochrane Library. [cited 2024 Jul 2]; Available from: https://www.cochranelibrary.com/cdsr/doi/10.1002/14651858.CD001751.pub3/full

13 Jo J, Lee SH. Heat therapy for primary dysmenorrhea: A systematic review and meta-analysis of its effects on pain relief and quality of life. *Sci Rep.* 2018 Nov 2;8(1):16252.

14 Akin MD, Weingand KW, Hengehold DA, Goodale MB, Hinkle RT, Smith RP. Continuous low-level topical heat in the treatment of dysmenorrhea. *Obstet Gynecol.* 2001 Mar;97(3):343–9.

15 Navvabi Rigi S, Kermansaravi F, Navidian A, Safabakhsh L, Safarzadeh A, Khazaian S, et al. Comparing the analgesic effect of heat patch containing iron chip and ibuprofen for primary dysmenorrhea: a randomized controlled trial. *BMC Women's Health.* 2012 Aug 22;12:25.

16 Oates J. The Effect of Yoga on Menstrual Disorders: A Systematic Review. *The Journal of Alternative and Complementary Medicine*. 2017 Jun;23(6):407–17.

17 Yang NY, Kim SD. Effects of a Yoga Program on Menstrual Cramps and Menstrual Distress in Undergraduate Students with Primary Dysmenorrhea: A Single-Blind, Randomized Controlled Trial. *The Journal of Alternative and Complementary Medicine*. 2016 Sep;22(9):732–8.

18 NICE Guideline. Amenorrhoea | CKS | NICE [Internet]. 2024 [cited 2024 Jul 2]. Available from: https://cks.nice.org.uk/topics/amenorrhoea/background-information/definition/

19 Gimunová M, Paulínyová A, Bernaciková M, Paludo AC. The Prevalence of Menstrual Cycle Disorders in Female Athletes from Different Sports Disciplines: A Rapid Review. *Int J Environ Res Public Health*. 2022 Oct 31;19(21):14243.

20 Camden Clinical Commissioning Group. Secondary Amenorrhoea/Oligomenorrhoea Pathway. 2017.

21 Camden Clinical Commissioning Group. Secondary Amenorrhoea/Oligomenorrhoea Pathway. 2017.

22 Mitra A, Verbakel JY, Kasaven LS, Tzafetas M, Grewal K, Jones B, et al. The menstrual cycle and the COVID-19 pandemic. *PLoS One*. 2023 Oct 11;18(10):e0290413.

23 Gao M, Zhang H, Gao Z, Cheng X, Sun Y, Qiao M, et al. Global and regional prevalence and burden for premenstrual syndrome and premenstrual dysphoric disorder. *Medicine* (Baltimore). 2022 Jan 7;101(1):e28528.

24 Mitra A, Verbakel JY, Kasaven LS, Tzafetas M, Grewal K, Jones B, et al. The menstrual cycle and the COVID-19 pandemic. *PLoS One*. 2023 Oct 11;18(10):e0290413.

Your cycle, start to finish

1 Amy E. Lacroix; Hurria Gondal; Karlie R. Shumway; Michelle D. Langaker. Physiology, Menarche https://www.ncbi.nlm.nih.gov/books/NBK470216/

2 Gudipally PR, Sharma GK. Premenstrual Syndrome. In: StatPearls [Internet]. Treasure Island (FL): StatPearls Publishing; 2024 [cited 2024 Oct 13]. Available from: http://www.ncbi.nlm.nih.gov/books/NBK560698/

3 Widholm O, Kantero RL. A statistical analysis of the menstrual patterns of 8,000 Finnish girls and their mothers. *Acta Obstet Gynecol Scand Suppl.* 1971;14:Suppl 14:1-36.

4 World Health Organization. Eliminating female genital mutilation: an interagency statement – OHCHR, UNAIDS, UNDP, UNECA, UNESCO, UNFPA, UNHCR, UNICEF, UNIFEM, WHO. Eliminer les mutilations sexuelles féminines : déclaration interinstitutions HCDH, OMS, ONUSIDA, PNUD, UNCEA, UNESCO, UNFPA, UNCHR, UNICEF, UNIFEM [Internet]. 2008; Available from: https://apps.who.int/iris/handle/10665/43839

5 Hickey M, Balen A. Menstrual disorders in adolescence: investigation and management. *Human Reproduction Update.* 2003 Sep 1;9(5):493–504.

6 Hickey M, Balen A. Menstrual disorders in adolescence: investigation and management. *Human Reproduction Update.* 2003 Sep 1;9(5):493–504.

7 Chauhan G, Tadi P. Physiology, Postpartum Changes. In: StatPearls [Internet]. Treasure Island (FL): StatPearls Publishing; 2024 [cited 2024 Oct 13]. Available from: http://www.ncbi.nlm.nih.gov/books/NBK555904/

8 NHS. nhs.uk. 2020 [cited 2024 Oct 13]. Your body after the birth. Available from: https://www.nhs.uk/pregnancy/labour-and-birth/after-the-birth/your-body/

9 Crowley WR. Neuroendocrine regulation of lactation and milk production. *Compr Physiol.* 2015 Jan;5(1):255–91.

10 World Health Organization. The World Health Organization Multinational Study of Breast-feeding and Lactational Amenorrhea. II. Factors associated with the length of amenorrhea. World Health Organization Task Force on Methods for the Natural Regulation of Fertility. Fertility and sterility [Internet]. 1998 Sep [cited 2024 Oct 13];70(3). Available from: https://pubmed.ncbi.nlm.nih.gov/9757874/

11 Campbell OM, Gray RH. Characteristics and determinants of postpartum ovarian function in women in the United States. *Am J Obstet Gynecol.* 1993 Jul;169(1):55–60.

12 Campino C, Ampuero S, Díaz S, Serón-Ferré M. Prolactin bioactivity and the duration of lactational amenorrhea. *J Clin Endocrinol Metab.* 1994 Oct;79(4):970–4.

13 Chauhan G, Tadi P. Physiology, Postpartum Changes. In: StatPearls [Internet]. Treasure Island (FL): StatPearls Publishing; 2024 [cited

2024 Oct 13]. Available from: http://www.ncbi.nlm.nih.gov/books/NB K555904/

14 University Hospital Bristol NFT. Post-birth contraception [Internet]. [cited 2024 Oct 13]. Available from: https://www.uhbristol.nhs.uk/ patients-and-visitors/your-hospitals/st-michaels-hospital/what-we-do/ midwifery-services/post-birth-contraception/lactational-amenorrhea-method-(lam)/

15 Haufe A, Baker FC, Leeners B. The role of ovarian hormones in the pathophysiology of perimenopausal sleep disturbances: A systematic review. *Sleep Medicine Reviews*. 2022 Dec 1;66:101710.

16 Hello Period. Hello Period. [cited 2024 Oct 13]. Menstrual Disc vs Cup: Which is Better? 8 Key Differences. Available from: https:// helloperiod.com/blogs/menstrual-cup-articles-and-blog/ the-6-key-differences-between-menstrual-cups-and-menstrual-discs

17 DeLoughery E, Colwill AC, Edelman A, Samuelson Bannow B. Red blood cell capacity of modern menstrual products: considerations for assessing heavy menstrual bleeding. *BMJ Sex Reprod Health*. 2024 Jan 9;50(1):21–6.

18 Hello Period. Hello Period. [cited 2024 Oct 13]. Menstrual Disc vs Cup: Which is Better? 8 Key Differences. Available from: https:// helloperiod.com/blogs/menstrual-cup-articles-and-blog/ the-6-key-differences-between-menstrual-cups-and-menstrual-discs

19 Hello Period. Hello Period. [cited 2024 Oct 13]. Menstrual Disc vs Cup: Which is Better? 8 Key Differences. Available from: https:// helloperiod.com/blogs/menstrual-cup-articles-and-blog/ the-6-key-differences-between-menstrual-cups-and-menstrual-discs

20 Hello Period. Hello Period. [cited 2024 Oct 13]. Menstrual Disc vs Cup: Which is Better? 8 Key Differences. Available from: https://helloperiod. com/blogs/menstrual-cup-articles-and-blog/ the-6-key-differences-between-menstrual-cups-and-menstrual-discs

21 Bowman N, Thwaites A. Menstrual cup and risk of IUD expulsion – a systematic review. *Contraception and Reproductive Medicine*. 2023 Jan 21;8(1):15.

Contraception

1 ActionAid UK. UK Period poverty rises from 12 to 21% | ActionAid UK. [cited 2024 Oct 13]. Available from: https://www.actionaid.org.uk/blog/2023/05/26/cost-living-uk-period-poverty-risen

2 United Nations. Contraceptive Use by Method 2019: Data Booklet. UN; 2019 [cited 2024 Jul 2]. Available from: https://www.un-ilibrary.org/content/books/9789210046527

3 United Nations. Contraceptive Use by Method 2019: Data Booklet. UN; 2019 [cited 2024 Jul 2]. Available from: https://www.un-ilibrary.org/content/books/9789210046527

4 United Nations. Contraceptive Use by Method 2019: Data Booklet. UN; 2019 [cited 2024 Jul 2]. Available from: https://www.un-ilibrary.org/content/books/9789210046527

5 Khan F, Mukhtar S, Dickinson IK, Sriprasad S. The story of the condom. *Indian J Urol.* 2013;29(1):12–5.

6 Khan F, Mukhtar S, Dickinson IK, Sriprasad S. The story of the condom. *Indian J Urol.* 2013;29(1):12–5.

7 Liao PV, Dollin J. Half a century of the oral contraceptive pill. *Can Fam Physician.* 2012 Dec;58(12):e757–60.

8 Liao PV, Dollin J. Half a century of the oral contraceptive pill. *Can Fam Physician.* 2012 Dec;58(12):e757–60.

9 Liao PV, Dollin J. Half a century of the oral contraceptive pill. *Can Fam Physician.* 2012 Dec;58(12):e757–60.

10 Le Guen M, Schantz C, Régnier-Loilier A, de La Rochebrochard E. Reasons for rejecting hormonal contraception in Western countries: A systematic review. *Social Science & Medicine.* 2021 Sep 1;284:114247.

11 Fakhri N, Chad MA, Lahkim M, Houari A, Dehbi H, Belmouden A, et al. Risk factors for breast cancer in women: an update review. *Med Oncol.* 2022 Sep 7;39(12):197.

12 Yland JJ, Bresnick KA, Hatch EE, Wesselink AK, Mikkelsen EM, Rothman KJ, et al. Pregravid contraceptive use and fecundability: prospective cohort study. *BMJ.* 2020 Nov 11;371:m3966.

13 Allen RH. Combined estrogen-progestin oral contraceptives: Patient selection, counseling, and use. In: UpToDate. Wolters Kluwer; 2024.

14 Martell S, Marini C, Kondas CA, Deutch AB. Psychological side effects of hormonal contraception: a disconnect between patients and providers. *Contracept Reprod Med.* 2023 Jan 17;8:9.

15 Family Planning Association. Survey finds worrying gaps in GP contraceptive provision [Internet]. Family Planning Association. 2017 [cited 2024 Jul 2]. Available from: https://www.fpa.org.uk/survey-finds-worrying-gaps-in-gp-contraceptive-provision/

16 Contraception Choices. Withdrawal [Internet]. [cited 2024 Oct 13]. Available from: https://www.contraceptionchoices.org/FSRH/ContraceptionChoices/Contraception-Methods/Withdrawal.aspx

17 Duane M, Stanford JB, Porucznik CA, Vigil P. Fertility Awareness-Based Methods for Women's Health and Family Planning. *Front Med* (Lausanne). 2022 May 24;9:858977.

18 Hirschberg AL. Challenging Aspects of Research on the Influence of the Menstrual Cycle and Oral Contraceptives on Physical Performance. *Sports Med.* 2022 Jul;52(7):1453–6.

19 Milsom I, Korver T. Ovulation incidence with oral contraceptives: a literature review. *BMJ Sexual & Reproductive Health.* 2008 Oct 1;34(4): 237–46.

Part 2: Living Alongside Your Cycle

Nutrition

1 Benton MJ, Hutchins AM, Dawes JJ. Effect of menstrual cycle on resting metabolism: A systematic review and meta-analysis. *PLOS ONE.* 2020 Jul 13;15(7):e0236025.

2 Barr SI, Janelle KC, Prior JC. Energy intakes are higher during the luteal phase of ovulatory menstrual cycles. *Am J Clin Nutr.* 1995 Jan;61(1):39–43.

3 Rogan MM, Black KE. Dietary energy intake across the menstrual cycle: a narrative review. *Nutr Rev.* 2023 Jun 9;81(7):869–86.

4 Klump KL, Keel PK, Racine SE, Burt SA, Neale M, Sisk CL, et al. The interactive effects of estrogen and progesterone on changes in emotional eating across the menstrual cycle. *Journal of Abnormal Psychology.* 2013;122(1):131–7.

5 Edler C, Lipson SF, Keel PK. Ovarian hormones and binge eating in bulimia nervosa. *Psychological Medicine.* 2007 Jan;37(1):131–41.

6 Fowler N, Vo PT, Sisk CL, Klump KL. Stress as a potential moderator of ovarian hormone influences on binge eating in women. *F1000Res*. 2019 Feb 27;8:F1000 Faculty Rev-222.

7 Davidsen L, Vistisen B, Astrup A. Impact of the menstrual cycle on determinants of energy balance: a putative role in weight loss attempts. *Int J Obes* (Lond). 2007 Dec;31(12):1777–85.

8 Klump KL, Di Dio AM. Combined Oral Contraceptive Use and Risk for Binge Eating in Women: Potential Gene x Hormone Interactions. *Front Neuroendocrinol*. 2022 Oct;67:101039.

9 Davidsen L, Vistisen B, Astrup A. Impact of the menstrual cycle on determinants of energy balance: a putative role in weight loss attempts. *Int J Obes* (Lond). 2007 Dec;31(12):1777–85.

10 Hummel J, Benkendorff C, Fritsche L, Prystupa K, Vosseler A, Gancheva S, et al. Brain insulin action on peripheral insulin sensitivity in women depends on menstrual cycle phase. *Nat Metab*. 2023 Sep;5(9):1475–82.

11 Yeung EH, Zhang C, Mumford SL, Ye A, Trevisan M, Chen L, et al. Longitudinal Study of Insulin Resistance and Sex Hormones over the Menstrual Cycle: The BioCycle Study. *The Journal of Clinical Endocrinology & Metabolism*. 2010 Dec 1;95(12):5435–42.

12 MacGregor KA, Gallagher IJ, Moran CN. Relationship Between Insulin Sensitivity and Menstrual Cycle Is Modified by BMI, Fitness, and Physical Activity in NHANES. *J Clin Endocrinol Metab*. 2021 Jun 10;106(10):2979–90.

13 Tarnopolsky LJ, MacDougall JD, Atkinson SA, Tarnopolsky MA, Sutton JR. Gender differences in substrate for endurance exercise. *J Appl Physiol* (1985). 1990 Jan;68(1):302–8.

14 Tarnopolsky MA, Atkinson SA, Phillips SM, MacDougall JD. Carbohydrate loading and metabolism during exercise in men and women. *J Appl Physiol* (1985). 1995 Apr;78(4):1360–8.

15 Carter SL, Rennie C, Tarnopolsky MA. Substrate utilization during endurance exercise in men and women after endurance training. *Am J Physiol Endocrinol Metab*. 2001 Jun;280(6):E898-907.

16 Devries MC, Hamadeh MJ, Phillips SM, Tarnopolsky MA. Menstrual cycle phase and sex influence muscle glycogen utilization and glucose turnover during moderate-intensity endurance exercise. *Am J Physiol Regul Integr Comp Physiol*. 2006 Oct;291(4):R1120-1128.

17 Venables MC, Achten J, Jeukendrup AE. Determinants of fat oxidation during exercise in healthy men and women: a cross-sectional study. *J Appl Physiol* (1985). 2005 Jan;98(1):160–7.

18 Cano A, Ventura L, Martinez G, Cugusi L, Caria M, Deriu F, et al. Analysis of sex-based differences in energy substrate utilization during moderate-intensity aerobic exercise. *Eur J Appl Physiol.* 2022;122(1):29–70.

19 Kriengsinyos W, Wykes LJ, Goonewardene LA, Ball RO, Pencharz PB. Phase of menstrual cycle affects lysine requirement in healthy women. *Am J Physiol Endocrinol Metab.* 2004 Sep;287(3):E489-496.

20 Kalkhoff RK. Metabolic effects of progesterone. *Am J Obstet Gynecol.* 1982 Mar 15;142(6 Pt 2):735–8.

21 Tiller NB, Elliott-Sale KJ, Knechtle B, Wilson PB, Roberts JD, Millet GY. Do Sex Differences in Physiology Confer a Female Advantage in Ultra-Endurance Sport? *Sports Med.* 2021 May;51(5):895–915.

22 Lariviere F, Moussalli R, Garrel DR. Increased leucine flux and leucine oxidation during the luteal phase of the menstrual cycle in women. *Am J Physiol.* 1994 Sep;267(3 Pt 1):E422-428.

23 Sawai A, Tsuzuki K, Yamauchi M, Kimura N, Tsushima T, Sugiyama K, et al. The effects of estrogen and progesterone on plasma amino acids levels: evidence from change plasma amino acids levels during the menstrual cycle in women. *Biological Rhythm Research.* 2020 Jan 2;51(1):151–64.

24 Bernstein MT, Graff LA, Avery L, Palatnick C, Parnerowski K, Targownik LE. Gastrointestinal symptoms before and during menses in healthy women. *BMC Women's Health.* 2014 Jan 22;14:14.

25 Houghton LA, Lea R, Jackson N, Whorwell PJ. The menstrual cycle affects rectal sensitivity in patients with irritable bowel syndrome but not healthy volunteers. *Gut.* 2002 Apr 1;50(4):471–4.

26 Pati GK, Kar C, Narayan J, Uthansingh K, Behera M, Sahu MK, et al. Irritable Bowel Syndrome and the Menstrual Cycle. *Cureus.* 13(1):e12692.

27 Bernstein MT, Graff LA, Avery L, Palatnick C, Parnerowski K, Targownik LE. Gastrointestinal symptoms before and during menses in healthy women. *BMC Womens Health.* 2014 Jan 22;14:14.

28 Agata Mulak YT, Muriel Larauche. Sex hormones in the modulation of irritable bowel syndrome. *World Journal of Gastroenterology.* 2014 Mar 14;20(10):2433–48.

29 Dajani EZ, Shahwan TG, Dajani NE. Prostaglandins and brain-gut axis. *J Physiol Pharmacol.* 2003 Dec;54 Suppl 4:155–64.

30 Agata Mulak YT, Muriel Larauche. Sex hormones in the modulation of irritable bowel syndrome. *World Journal of Gastroenterology*. 2014 Mar 14;20(10):2433–48.

31 Baker JM, Al-Nakkash L, Herbst-Kralovetz MM. Estrogen-gut microbiome axis: Physiological and clinical implications. *Maturitas*. 2017 Sep;103:45–53.

32 Shin JH, Park YH, Sim M, Kim SA, Joung H, Shin DM. Serum level of sex steroid hormone is associated with diversity and profiles of human gut microbiome. *Res Microbiol*. 2019;170(4–5):192–201.

33 Baker JM, Al-Nakkash L, Herbst-Kralovetz MM. Estrogen-gut microbiome axis: Physiological and clinical implications. *Maturitas*. 2017 Sep;103:45–53.

34 Bernstein MT, Graff LA, Avery L, Palatnick C, Parnerowski K, Targownik LE. Gastrointestinal symptoms before and during menses in healthy women. *BMC Womens Health*. 2014 Jan 22;14:14.

35 Fahrenholtz IL, Sjödin A, Benardot D, Tornberg ÅB, Skouby S, Faber J, et al. Within-day energy deficiency and reproductive function in female endurance athletes. *Scand J Med Sci Sports*. 2018 Mar;28(3):1139–46.

36 Benardot D. Energy Thermodynamics Revisited: Energy Intake Strategies for Optimizing Athlete Body Composition and Performance. *Journal of Exercise Science and Health*. 2013 Dec 18;11:1–13.

37 Blumberg J, Hahn SL, Bakke J. Intermittent fasting: consider the risks of disordered eating for your patient. *Clinical Diabetes and Endocrinology*. 2023 Oct 21;9(1):4.

Bodyweight and the menstrual cycle

1 Reavey JJ, Walker C, Murray AA, Brito-Mutunayagam S, Sweeney S, Nicol M, et al. Obesity is associated with heavy menstruation that may be due to delayed endometrial repair. *J Endocrinol*. 2021 Mar 9;249(2):71–82.

2 Wei S, Schmidt MD, Dwyer T, Norman RJ, Venn AJ. Obesity and menstrual irregularity: associations with SHBG, testosterone, and insulin. *Obesity* (Silver Spring). 2009 May;17(5):1070–6.

3 Ko KM, Han K, Chung YJ, Yoon KH, Park YG, Lee SH. Association between Body Weight Changes and Menstrual Irregularity: The Korea National Health and Nutrition Examination Survey 2010 to 2012. *Endocrinol Metab* (Seoul). 2017 Jun;32(2):248–56.

4 Teede H, Deeks A, Moran L. Polycystic ovary syndrome: a complex condition with psychological, reproductive and metabolic manifestations that impacts on health across the lifespan. *BMC Med.* 2010 Jun 30;8:41.

5 Lee I, Cooney LG, Saini S, Sammel MD, Allison KC, Dokras A. Increased odds of disordered eating in polycystic ovary syndrome: a systematic review and meta-analysis. *Eat Weight Disord.* 2019 Oct;24(5):787–97.

6 Qin H, Lin Z, Vásquez E, Luan X, Guo F, Xu L. Association between obesity and the risk of uterine fibroids: a systematic review and meta-analysis. *J Epidemiol Community Health.* 2021 Feb;75(2):197–204.

7 Hassan MAM, Killick SR. Negative lifestyle is associated with a significant reduction in fecundity. *Fertility and Sterility.* 2004 Feb 1;81(2):384–92.

8 Bombak AE, McPhail D, Ward P. Reproducing stigma: Interpreting 'overweight' and 'obese' women's experiences of weight-based discrimination in reproductive healthcare. *Social Science & Medicine.* 2016 Oct 1;166:94–101.

9 Phelan SM, Burgess DJ, Yeazel MW, Hellerstedt WL, Griffin JM, van Ryn M. Impact of weight bias and stigma on quality of care and outcomes for patients with obesity. *Obes Rev.* 2015 Apr;16(4):319–26.

10 Vaillancourt S, Moore G. Fat Stigma in Women's Health. *The Journal for Nurse Practitioners.* 2019 Feb 1;15(2):207–8.

11 Bertone-Johnson ER, Ronnenberg AG, Houghton SC, Nobles C, Zagarins SE, Takashima-Uebelhoer BB, et al. Association of inflammation markers with menstrual symptom severity and premenstrual syndrome in young women. *Hum Reprod.* 2014 Sep;29(9):1987–94.

12 Saei Ghare Naz M, Kiani Z, Rashidi Fakari F, Ghasemi V, Abed M, Ozgoli G. The Effect of Micronutrients on Pain Management of Primary Dysmenorrhea: a Systematic Review and Meta-Analysis. *J Caring Sci.* 2020 Mar 1;9(1):47–56.

13 Snipe RMJ, Brelis B, Kappas C, Young JK, Eishold L, Chui JM, et al. Omega-3 long chain polyunsaturated fatty acids as a potential treatment for reducing dysmenorrhoea pain: Systematic literature review and meta-analysis. *Nutrition & Dietetics.* 2024;81(1):94–106.

14 Rahbar N, Asgharzadeh N, Ghorbani R. Effect of omega-3 fatty acids on intensity of primary dysmenorrhea. *International Journal of Gynecology & Obstetrics.* 2012;117(1):45–7.

15 Snipe RMJ, Brelis B, Kappas C, Young JK, Eishold L, Chui JM, et al. Omega-3 long chain polyunsaturated fatty acids as a potential treatment

for reducing dysmenorrhoea pain: Systematic literature review and meta-analysis. *Nutrition & Dietetics.* 2024;81(1):94–106.

16 Heart UK TCC. Omega 3 fats [Internet]. [cited 2024 Jun 28]. Available from: https://www.heartuk.org.uk/low-cholesterol-foods/omega-3-fats

17 BDA TA of UD. Omega-3 [Internet]. [cited 2024 Jun 28]. Available from: https://www.bda.uk.com/resource/omega-3.html

18 Mohammad-Alizadeh Charandabi S, Mirghafourvand M, Nezamivand-Chegini S, Javadzadeh Y. Calcium With and Without Magnesium for Primary Dysmenorrhea: A Double-Blind Randomized PlaceboControlled Trial. *International Journal of Women's Health and Reproduction Sciences.* 2017 Apr 28;5(4):332–8.

19 Zarei S, Mohammad-Alizadeh-Charandabi S, Mirghafourvand M, Javadzadeh Y, Effati-Daryani F. Effects of Calcium-Vitamin D and Calcium-Alone on Pain Intensity and Menstrual Blood Loss in Women with Primary Dysmenorrhea: A Randomized Controlled Trial. *Pain Med.* 2017 Jan 1;18(1):3–13.

20 Abdi F, Amjadi MA, Zaheri F, Rahnemaei FA. Role of vitamin D and calcium in the relief of primary dysmenorrhea: a systematic review. *Obstet Gynecol Sci.* 2021 Jan;64(1):13–26.

21 Zarei S, Mohammad-Alizadeh-Charandabi S, Mirghafourvand M, Javadzadeh Y, Effati-Daryani F. Effects of Calcium-Vitamin D and Calcium-Alone on Pain Intensity and Menstrual Blood Loss in Women with Primary Dysmenorrhea: A Randomized Controlled Trial. *Pain Med.* 2017 Jan 1;18(1):3–13.

22 Yaralizadeh M, Nezamivand-Chegini S, Najar S, Namjoyan F, Abedi P. Effectiveness of Magnesium on Menstrual Symptoms Among Dysmenorrheal College Students: A Randomized Controlled Trial. *NaN.* 2024;(2):70–6.

23 Proctor M, Murphy PA. Herbal and dietary therapies for primary and secondary dysmenorrhoea – Proctor, M – 2001 | Cochrane Library.

24 Yaralizadeh M, Nezamivand-Chegini S, Najar S, Namjoyan F, Abedi P. Effectiveness of Magnesium on Menstrual Symptoms Among Dysmenorrheal College Students: A Randomized Controlled Trial. *NaN.* 2024;(2):70–6.

25 Proctor M, Murphy PA. Herbal and dietary therapies for primary and secondary dysmenorrhoea – Proctor, M – 2001 | Cochrane Library.

26 Gök S, Gök B. Investigation of Laboratory and Clinical Features of Primary Dysmenorrhea: Comparison of Magnesium and Oral Contraceptives in Treatment. *Cureus*. 14(11):e32028.

27 Obiagwu HI, Eleje GU, Obiechina NJA, Nwosu BO, Udigwe GO, Ikechebelu JI, et al. Efficacy of zinc supplementation for the treatment of dysmenorrhoea: a double-blind randomised controlled trial. *J Int Med Res*. 2023 May 10;51(5):03000605231171489.

28 Sangestani G, Khatiban M, Marci R, Piva I. The Positive Effects of Zinc Supplements on the Improvement of Primary Dysmenorrhea and Premenstrual Symptoms: A Double-blind, Randomized, Controlled Trial. *Journal of Midwifery and Reproductive Health*. 2015 Jul 1;3(3):378–84.

29 Kashefi F, Khajehei M, Tabatabaeichehr M, Alavinia M, Asili J. Comparison of the Effect of Ginger and Zinc Sulfate on Primary Dysmenorrhea: A Placebo-Controlled Randomized Trial. *Pain Management Nursing*. 2014 Dec 1;15(4):826–33.

30 Teimoori B, Ghasemi M, Hoseini ZSA, Razavi M. The Efficacy of Zinc Administration in the Treatment of Primary Dysmenorrhea. *Oman Med J*. 2016 Mar;31(2):107–11.

31 Rabinovich D, Smadi Y. Zinc. In: StatPearls [Internet]. Treasure Island (FL): StatPearls Publishing; 2024 [cited 2024 Jun 28]. Available from: http://www.ncbi.nlm.nih.gov/books/NBK547698/

32 Khayat S, Fanaei H, Kheirkhah M, Moghadam ZB, Kasaeian A, Javadimehr M. Curcumin attenuates severity of premenstrual syndrome symptoms: A randomized, double-blind, placebo-controlled trial. *Complement Ther Med*. 2015 Jun;23(3):318–24.

33 Sharifipour F, Siahkal SF, Qaderi K, Mohaghegh Z, Zahedian M, Azizi F. Effect of Curcumin on Dysmenorrhea and Symptoms of Premenstrual Syndrome: A Systematic Review and Meta-Analysis. *Korean J Fam Med*. 2024 Mar;45(2):96–104.

34 Rahman SF, Hardi GW, Maras MAJ, Riva YR. Influence of Curcumin and Ginger in Primary Dysmenorrhea: A Review. *International Journal of Applied Engineering Research*. 15(7):634–8.

35 Khayat S, Kheirkhah M, Fanaei H, Behboodi Moghadam Z, Pourmohsen M, Kasaeiyan A. Comparison the effects of Ginger and Curcumin in treatment of premenstrual syndrome. *Iranian South Medical Journal*. 2015 Jul 4;18(3):575–86.

36 Hesami S, Kavianpour M, Rashidi Nooshabadi M, Yousefi M, Lalooha F, Khadem Haghighian H. Randomized, double-blind, placebo-controlled clinical trial studying the effects of Turmeric in combination with mefenamic acid in patients with primary dysmenorrhoea. *J Gynecol Obstet Hum Reprod.* 2021 Apr;50(4):101840.

37 Hewlings SJ, Kalman DS. Curcumin: A Review of Its' Effects on Human Health. *Foods.* 2017 Oct 22;6(10):92.

38 Palmery M, Saraceno A, Vaiarelli A, Carlomagno G. Oral contraceptives and changes in nutritional requirements. *Eur Rev Med Pharmacol Sci.* 2013 Jul;17(13):1804–13.

39 Hudiburgh NK, Milner AN. Influence of oral contraceptives on ascorbic acid and triglyceride status. *J Am Diet Assoc.* 1979 Jul;75(1):19–22.

40 Hameed A, Majeed T, Rauf S, Ashraf M, Jalil MA, Nasrullah M, et al. Effect of oral and injectable contraceptives on serum calcium, magnesium and phosphorus in women. *J Ayub Med Coll Abbottabad.* 2001;13(3):24–5.

Movement

1 Vertinsky P. Exercise, Physical Capability, and the Eternally Wounded Woman in Late Nineteenth Century North America. *Journal of Sport History.* 1987;14(1):7–27.

2 Wellcome Collection. Wellcome Collection. 2017 [cited 2024 Jul 6]. The law of periodicity for menstruation. Available from: https://wellcome collection.org/articles/We9i3h4AAA5amHVO

3 Wellcome Collection. Wellcome Collection. 2017 [cited 2024 Jul 6]. The law of periodicity for menstruation. Available from: https://wellcomecol lection.org/articles/We9i3h4AAA5amHVO

4 Jacobi MP. *The question of rest for women during menstruation* [Internet]. New York: G.P. Putnam's Sons; 1877 [cited 2024 Jul 6]. p. 286 Available from: http://archive.org/details/questionofrestfo00jacoiala

5 Buell J. An analysis of restrictions and their negative effects on women's running. The University of Texas at Austin; 2020.

6 Blount C. The History of Gender Discrimination in Women's Distance Running: Long-term Consequences and Solutions. Academic Festival [Internet]. 2022 Apr 29; Available from: https://digitalcommons.sacred-heart.edu/acadfest/2022/all/10

7 The Sports Museum. The Sports Museum. 2024 [cited 2024 Jul 6]. Bobbi Gibb Marathon Pioneer. Available from: https://www.sportsmuseum.org/curators-corner/bobbi-gibb-marathon-pioneer/

8 Butler C. *Runner's World*. 2018 [cited 2024 Jul 6]. Sole Sisters of '72. Available from: https://www.runnersworld.com/runners-stories/a20966306/sole-sisters-of-72/

9 Guthold R, Stevens GA, Riley LM, Bull FC. Worldwide trends in insufficient physical activity from 2001 to 2016: a pooled analysis of 358 population-based surveys with 1·9 million participants. *The Lancet Global Health*. 2018 Oct 1;6(10):e1077–86.

10 Peng B, Ng JYY, Ha AS. Barriers and facilitators to physical activity for young adult women: a systematic review and thematic synthesis of qualitative literature. *International Journal of Behavioral Nutrition and Physical Activity*. 2023 Feb 27;20(1):23.

11 World Health Organization. 2024 [cited 2024 Jul 6]. Physical activity. Available from: https://www.who.int/news-room/fact-sheets/detail/physical-activity

12 Sport England. Sport England. [cited 2024 Jul 6]. Gender. Available from: https://www.sportengland.org/research-and-data/research/gender

13 Elgaddal N, Kramarow E, Reuben C. Physical Activity Among Adults Aged 18 and Over: United States, 2020. *NCHS Data Brief*. 2022;(443).

14 Nuffield Health. Nuffield Health. 2023 [cited 2024 Jul 6]. Periods are making it harder for 84% of teenage girls to take part in sports and fitness. Available from: https://www.nuffieldhealth.com/article/menstrual-cycle-impact-on-physical-activity

15 Guardian Sport. Wimbledon will allow dark undershorts due to female players' period concerns. *The Guardian* [Internet]. 2022 Nov 17 [cited 2024 Jul 6]; Available from: https://www.theguardian.com/sport/2022/nov/17/wimbledon-allow-dark-undershorts-due-to-female-players-period-concerns-tennis

16 Taylor L. England Lionesses switch to blue shorts after players voice period concerns. *The Guardian* [Internet]. 2023 Apr 3 [cited 2024 Jul 6]; Available from: https://www.theguardian.com/football/2023/apr/03/england-lionesses-new-kit-blue-shorts-player-period-concerns

17 McNulty KL, Ansdell P, Goodall S, Thomas K, Elliott-Sale KJ, Howatson G, et al. The Symptoms Experienced by Naturally Menstruating Women and Oral Contraceptive Pill Users and Their Perceived Effects on Exercise

Performance and Recovery Time Posttraining. *Women in Sport and Physical Activity Journal.* 2024 Jan 1;32(1).

18 McNulty KL, Ansdell P, Goodall S, Thomas K, Elliott-Sale KJ, Howatson G, et al. The Symptoms Experienced by Naturally Menstruating Women and Oral Contraceptive Pill Users and Their Perceived Effects on Exercise Performance and Recovery Time Posttraining. *Women in Sport and Physical Activity Journal.* 2024 Jan 1;32(1).

19 Carmichael MA, Thomson RL, Moran LJ, Wycherley TP. The Impact of Menstrual Cycle Phase on Athletes' Performance: A Narrative Review. *International Journal of Environmental Research and Public Health.* 2021 Jan;18(4):1667.

20 Bharati M. Comparing the Effects of Yoga & Oral Calcium Administration in Alleviating Symptoms of Premenstrual Syndrome in Medical Undergraduates. *J Caring Sci.* 2016 Sep;5(3):179–85.

21 El-Lithy A, El-Mazny A, Sabbour A, El-Deeb A. Effect of aerobic exercise on premenstrual symptoms, haematological and hormonal parameters in young women. *J Obstet Gynaecol.* 2015 May;35(4):389–92.

22 Petersen AMW, Pedersen BK. The anti-inflammatory effect of exercise. *J Appl Physiol* (1985). 2005 Apr;98(4):1154–62.

23 Tsai SY. Effect of Yoga Exercise on Premenstrual Symptoms among Female Employees in Taiwan. *Int J Environ Res Public Health.* 2016 Jul;13(7):721.

24 Vaghela N, Mishra D, Sheth M, Dani VB. To compare the effects of aerobic exercise and yoga on Premenstrual syndrome. *J Educ Health Promot.* 2019;8:199.

25 McNamara A, Harris R, Minahan C. 'That time of the month' . . . for the biggest event of your career! Perception of menstrual cycle on performance of Australian athletes training for the 2020 Olympic and Paralympic Games. *BMJ Open Sport Exerc Med.* 2022;8(2):e001300.

26 McNulty KL, Elliott-Sale KJ, Dolan E, Swinton PA, Ansdell P, Goodall S, et al. The Effects of Menstrual Cycle Phase on Exercise Performance in Eumenorrheic Women: A Systematic Review and Meta-Analysis. *Sports Med.* 2020 Oct;50(10):1813–27.

27 McNulty KL, Elliott-Sale KJ, Dolan E, Swinton PA, Ansdell P, Goodall S, et al. The Effects of Menstrual Cycle Phase on Exercise Performance in Eumenorrheic Women: A Systematic Review and Meta-Analysis. *Sports Med.* 2020 Oct;50(10):1813–27.

28 Carmichael MA, Thomson RL, Moran LJ, Wycherley TP. The Impact of Menstrual Cycle Phase on Athletes' Performance: A Narrative Review. *International Journal of Environmental Research and Public Health.* 2021 Jan;18(4):1667.

29 Delp M, Chesbro GA, Pribble BA, Miller RM, Pereira HM, Black CD, et al. Higher rating of perceived exertion and lower perceived recovery following a graded exercise test during menses compared to non-bleeding days in untrained females. *Front Physiol.* 2024 Jan 11;14:1297242.

30 Romero-Parra N, Cupeiro R, Alfaro-Magallanes VM, Rael B, Rubio-Arias JÁ, Peinado AB, et al. Exercise-Induced Muscle Damage During the Menstrual Cycle: A Systematic Review and Meta-Analysis. *The Journal of Strength & Conditioning Research.* 2021 Feb;35(2):549.

31 Kannan P, Cheung KK, Lau BWM. Does aerobic exercise induced-analgesia occur through hormone and inflammatory cytokine-mediated mechanisms in primary dysmenorrhea? *Medical Hypotheses.* 2019 Feb 1;123:50–4.

32 Armour M, Ee CC, Naidoo D, Ayati Z, Chalmers KJ, Steel KA, et al. Exercise for dysmenorrhoea. *Cochrane Database Syst Rev.* 2019 Sep 20;9(9):CD004142.

33 Armour M, Ee CC, Naidoo D, Ayati Z, Chalmers KJ, Steel KA, et al. Exercise for dysmenorrhoea. *Cochrane Database Syst Rev.* 2019 Sep 20;9(9):CD004142.

34 Tsai IC, Hsu CW, Chang CH, Lei WT, Tseng PT, Chang KV. Comparative Effectiveness of Different Exercises for Reducing Pain Intensity in Primary Dysmenorrhea: A Systematic Review and Network Meta-analysis of Randomized Controlled Trials. *Sports Medicine – Open.* 2024 May 30;10(1):63.

35 Kanchibhotla D, Subramanian S, Singh D. Management of dysmenorrhea through yoga: A narrative review. *Front Pain Res* (Lausanne). 2023 Mar 30;4:1107669.

36 Kanchibhotla D, Subramanian S, Singh D. Management of dysmenorrhea through yoga: A narrative review. *Front Pain Res* (Lausanne). 2023 Mar 30;4:1107669.

37 Lowe DA, Baltgalvis KA, Greising SM. Mechanisms behind Estrogens' Beneficial Effect on Muscle Strength in Females. *Exerc Sport Sci Rev.* 2010 Apr;38(2):61–7.

38 Knowles OE, Aisbett B, Main LC, Drinkwater EJ, Orellana L, Lamon S. Resistance Training and Skeletal Muscle Protein Metabolism in Eumenorrheic Females: Implications for Researchers and Practitioners. *Sports Med.* 2019 Nov;49(11):1637–50.

39 Carmichael MA, Thomson RL, Moran LJ, Wycherley TP. The Impact of Menstrual Cycle Phase on Athletes' Performance: A Narrative Review. *International Journal of Environmental Research and Public Health.* 2021 Jan;18(4):1667.

40 Knowles OE, Aisbett B, Main LC, Drinkwater EJ, Orellana L, Lamon S. Resistance Training and Skeletal Muscle Protein Metabolism in Eumenorrheic Females: Implications for Researchers and Practitioners. *Sports Med.* 2019 Nov;49(11):1637–50.

41 Wikström-Frisén L, Boraxbekk CJ, Henriksson-Larsén K. Effects on power, strength and lean body mass of menstrual/oral contraceptive cycle based resistance training. *J Sports Med Phys Fitness.* 2017;57 (1–2):43–52.

42 Sung E, Han A, Hinrichs T, Vorgerd M, Manchado C, Platen P. Effects of follicular versus luteal phase-based strength training in young women. *Springerplus.* 2014 Nov 11;3:668.

43 Reis E, Frick U, Schmidtbleicher D. Frequency variations of strength training sessions triggered by the phases of the menstrual cycle. *Int J Sports Med.* 1995 Nov;16(8):545–50.

44 Kissow J, Jacobsen KJ, Gunnarsson TP, Jessen S, Hostrup M. Effects of Follicular and Luteal Phase-Based Menstrual Cycle Resistance Training on Muscle Strength and Mass. *Sports Med.* 2022 Dec;52(12):2813–9.

45 Cook CJ, Kilduff LP, Crewther BT. Basal and stress-induced salivary testosterone variation across the menstrual cycle and linkage to motivation and muscle power. *Scand J Med Sci Sports.* 2018 Apr;28(4):1345–53.

46 Bateup HS, Booth A, Shirtcliff EA, Granger DA. Testosterone, cortisol, and women's competition. *Evolution and Human Behavior.* 2002 May;23(3):181–92.

47 Blagrove RC, Bruinvels G, Pedlar CR. Variations in strength-related measures during the menstrual cycle in eumenorrheic women: A systematic review and meta-analysis. *J Sci Med Sport.* 2020 Dec;23(12): 1220–7.

48 Colenso-Semple LM, D'Souza AC, Elliott-Sale KJ, Phillips SM. Current evidence shows no influence of women's menstrual cycle phase on acute

strength performance or adaptations to resistance exercise training. *Front Sports Act Living.* 2023 Mar 23;5:1054542.

49 Colenso-Semple LM, D'Souza AC, Elliott-Sale KJ, Phillips SM. Current evidence shows no influence of women's menstrual cycle phase on acute strength performance or adaptations to resistance exercise training. *Front Sports Act Living.* 2023 Mar 23;5:1054542.

50 Elliott-Sale KJ, Minahan CL, de Jonge XAKJ, Ackerman KE, Sipilä S, Constantini NW, et al. Methodological Considerations for Studies in Sport and Exercise Science with Women as Participants: A Working Guide for Standards of Practice for Research on Women. *Sports Med.* 2021;51(5):843–61.

51 Alzueta E, Zambotti M de, Javitz H, Dulai T, Albinni B, Simon KC, et al. Tracking Sleep, Temperature, Heart Rate, and Daily Symptoms Across the Menstrual Cycle with the Oura Ring in Healthy Women. *IJWH.* 2022 Apr 8;14:491–503.

52 Horvath SM, Drinkwater BL. Thermoregulation and the menstrual cycle. *Aviat Space Environ Med.* 1982 Aug 1;53(8):790–4.

53 Goldsmith E, Glaister M. The effect of the menstrual cycle on running economy. *J Sports Med Phys Fitness.* 2020 Apr;60(4):610–7.

54 Williams TJ, Krahenbuhl GS. Menstrual cycle phase and running economy. *Med Sci Sports Exerc.* 1997 Dec;29(12):1609–18.

55 Janse de Jonge XAK. Effects of the menstrual cycle on exercise performance. *Sports Med.* 2003;33(11):833–51.

56 Goldsmith E, Glaister M. The effect of the menstrual cycle on running economy. *J Sports Med Phys Fitness.* 2020 Apr;60(4):610–7.

57 Julian R, Hecksteden A, Fullagar HHK, Meyer T. The effects of menstrual cycle phase on physical performance in female soccer players. *PLOS ONE.* 2017 Mar 13;12(3):e0173951.

58 Greenhall M, Taipale RS, Ihalainen JK, Hackney AC. Influence of the Menstrual Cycle Phase on Marathon Performance in Recreational Runners. 2020 Aug 10 [cited 2024 Jul 6]; Available from: https://journals. humankinetics.com/view/journals/ijspp/16/4/article-p601.xml

59 Schmalenberger KM, Eisenlohr-Moul TA, Würth L, Schneider E, Thayer JF, Ditzen B, et al. A Systematic Review and Meta-Analysis of Within-Person Changes in Cardiac Vagal Activity across the Menstrual Cycle: Implications for Female Health and Future Studies. *J Clin Med.* 2019 Nov 12;8(11):1946.

60 Sims ST, Ware L, Capodilupo ER. Patterns of endogenous and exogenous ovarian hormone modulation on recovery metrics across the menstrual cycle. *BMJ Open Sport Exerc Med.* 2021;7(3):e001047.

61 Pearce E, Jolly K, Jones LL, Matthewman G, Zanganeh M, Daley A. Exercise for premenstrual syndrome: a systematic review and meta-analysis of randomised controlled trials. *BJGP Open.* 4(3):bjgpopen20X101032.

62 Yesildere Saglam H, Orsal O. Effect of exercise on premenstrual symptoms: A systematic review. *Complement Ther Med.* 2020 Jan;48:102272.

63 Elliott-Sale KJ, McNulty KL, Ansdell P, Goodall S, Hicks KM, Thomas K, et al. The Effects of Oral Contraceptives on Exercise Performance in Women: A Systematic Review and Meta-analysis. *Sports Med.* 2020;50(10):1785–812.

64 Elliott-Sale KJ, McNulty KL, Ansdell P, Goodall S, Hicks KM, Thomas K, et al. The Effects of Oral Contraceptives on Exercise Performance in Women: A Systematic Review and Meta-analysis. *Sports Med.* 2020;50(10):1785–812.

65 Nolan D, McNulty KL, Manninen M, Egan B. The Effect of Hormonal Contraceptive Use on Skeletal Muscle Hypertrophy, Power and Strength Adaptations to Resistance Exercise Training: A Systematic Review and Multilevel Meta-analysis. *Sports Med.* 2024 Jan;54(1):105–25.

66 Glenner-Frandsen A, With C, Gunnarsson TP, Hostrup M. The Effect of Monophasic Oral Contraceptives on Muscle Strength and Markers of Recovery After Exercise-Induced Muscle Damage: A Systematic Review. *Sports Health.* 2022 Sep 25;15(3):318–27.

67 Sanchez BN, Kraemer WJ, Maresh CM. Premenstrual Syndrome and Exercise: A Narrative Review. *Women.* 2023 Jun;3(2):348–64.

68 De Souza MJ, Toombs RJ, Scheid JL, O'Donnell E, West SL, Williams NI. High prevalence of subtle and severe menstrual disturbances in exercising women: confirmation using daily hormone measures. *Human Reproduction.* 2010 Feb 1;25(2):491–503.

69 Mountjoy M, Sundgot-Borgen J, Burke L, Carter S, Constantini N, Lebrun C, et al. The IOC consensus statement: beyond the Female Athlete Triad--Relative Energy Deficiency in Sport (RED-S). *Br J Sports Med.* 2014 Apr;48(7):491–7.

70 Mountjoy M, Sundgot-Borgen J, Burke L, Carter S, Constantini N, Lebrun C, et al. The IOC consensus statement: beyond the Female Athlete

Triad--Relative Energy Deficiency in Sport (RED-S). *Br J Sports Med.* 2014 Apr;48(7):491-7.

71 Mountjoy M, Sundgot-Borgen JK, Burke LM, Ackerman KE, Blauwet C, Constantini N, et al. IOC consensus statement on relative energy deficiency in sport (RED-S): 2018 update. *Br J Sports Med.* 2018 Jun 1;52(11):687-97.

72 Holtzman B, Ackerman KE. Recommendations and Nutritional Considerations for Female Athletes: Health and Performance. *Sports Med.* 2021;51(Suppl 1):43-57.

73 Pate RR, Miller BJ, Davis JM, Slentz CA, Klingshirn LA. Iron Status of Female Runners. *Int J Sport Nutr.* 1993 Jun 1;3(2):222-31.

Sleep

1 Lim AJR, Huang Z, Chua SE, Kramer MS, Yong EL. Sleep Duration, Exercise, Shift Work and Polycystic Ovarian Syndrome-Related Outcomes in a Healthy Population: A Cross-Sectional Study. *PLOS ONE.* 2016 Nov 21;11(11):e0167048.

2 Nam GE, Han K, Lee G. Association between sleep duration and menstrual cycle irregularity in Korean female adolescents. *Sleep Medicine.* 2017 Jul 1;35:62-6.

3 Jeon B, Baek J. Menstrual disturbances and its association with sleep disturbances: a systematic review. *BMC Womens Health.* 2023 Sep 1;23:470.

4 Sleep Foundation [Internet]. 2020 [cited 2024 Jun 23]. How To Determine Poor Sleep Quality. Available from: https://www.sleepfoundation.org/sleep-hygiene/how-to-determine-poor-quality-sleep

5 5 Stages of Sleep: Psychology, Cycle & Sequence [Internet]. 2023 [cited 2024 Jul 6]. Available from: https://www.simplypsychology.org/sleep-stages.html

6 Burgard SA, Ailshire JA. Gender and Time for Sleep among U.S. Adults. *Am Sociol Rev.* 2013 Feb;78(1):51-69.

7 Meers J, Stout-Aguilar J, Nowakowski S. Chapter 3 – Sex differences in sleep health. In: Grandner MA, editor. *Sleep and Health* [Internet]. Academic Press; 2019 [cited 2024 Jun 23]. p. 21-9. Available from: https://www.sciencedirect.com/science/article/pii/B9780128153734000034

8 Mong JA, Cusmano DM. Sex differences in sleep: impact of biological sex and sex steroids. *Philosophical Transactions of the Royal Society B: Biological Sciences.* 2016 Feb 19;371(1688):20150110.

9   Benge E, Pavlova M, Javaheri S. Sleep health challenges among women: insomnia across the lifespan. *Front Sleep* [Internet]. 2024 Feb 12 [cited 2024 Jun 23];3. Available from: https://www.frontiersin.org/articles/10.3389/frsle.2024.1322761

10 Li DX, Romans S, De Souza MJ, Murray B, Einstein G. Actigraphic and self-reported sleep quality in women: associations with ovarian hormones and mood. *Sleep Med. 2015 Oct;16(10):1217–24.*

11 de Zambotti M, Colrain IM, Baker FC. Interaction between reproductive hormones and physiological sleep in women. *J Clin Endocrinol Metab.* 2015 Apr;100(4):1426–33.

12 Freedman RR, Woodward S. Core body temperature during menopausal hot flushes. *Fertil Steril.* 1996 Jun;65(6):1141–4.

13 Eichling PS, Sahni J. Menopause related sleep disorders. *J Clin Sleep Med.* 2005 Jul 15;1(3):291–300.

14 Baker FC, Mitchell D, Driver HS. Oral contraceptives alter sleep and raise body temperature in young women. *Pflugers Arch.* 2001 Aug;442(5):729–37.

15 Li DX, Romans S, De Souza MJ, Murray B, Einstein G. Actigraphic and self-reported sleep quality in women: associations with ovarian hormones and mood. *Sleep Med.* 2015 Oct;16(10):1217–24.

16 Baker FC, Sassoon SA, Kahan T, Palaniappan L, Nicholas CL, Trinder J, et al. Perceived poor sleep quality in the absence of polysomnographic sleep disturbance in women with severe premenstrual syndrome. *Journal of Sleep Research.* 2012;21(5):535–45.

17 Reynolds WS, Fowke J, Dmochowski R. The Burden of Overactive Bladder on US Public Health. *Curr Bladder Dysfunct Rep.* 2016 Mar;11(1):8–13.

18 Weiss JP. Nocturia: focus on etiology and consequences. *Rev Urol.* 2012;14(3–4):48–55.

19 Burgard SA, Ailshire JA. Gender and Time for Sleep among U.S. Adults. *Am Sociol Rev.* 2013 Feb;78(1):51–69.

20 Baker FC, Lee KA. Menstrual Cycle Effects on Sleep. *Sleep Med Clin.* 2018 Sep;13(3):283–94.

21 Van Reen E, Kiesner J. Individual differences in self-reported difficulty sleeping across the menstrual cycle. *Arch Womens Ment Health.* 2016 Aug;19(4):599–608.

22 Driver HS, Werth E, Dijk DJ, Borbély AA. The Menstrual Cycle Effects on Sleep. *Sleep Medicine Clinics.* 2008 Mar 1;3(1):1–11.

23 Van Reen E, Kiesner J. Individual differences in self-reported difficulty sleeping across the menstrual cycle. *Arch Womens Ment Health.* 2016 Aug;19(4):599–608.

24 Baker FC, Driver HS, Rogers GG, Paiker J, Mitchell D. High nocturnal body temperatures and disturbedsleep in women with primary dysmenorrhea. *American Journal of Physiology-Endocrinology and Metabolism.* 1999 Dec;277(6):E1013–21.

25 Walker M. Why We Sleep: The New Science of Sleep and Dreams. Penguin UK; 2017. 419 p.

26 de Zambotti M, Willoughby AR, Sassoon SA, Colrain IM, Baker FC. Menstrual Cycle-Related Variation in Physiological Sleep in Women in the Early Menopausal Transition. *J Clin Endocrinol Metab.* 2015 Aug;100(8):2918–26.

27 de Zambotti M, Willoughby AR, Sassoon SA, Colrain IM, Baker FC. Menstrual Cycle-Related Variation in Physiological Sleep in Women in the Early Menopausal Transition. *J Clin Endocrinol Metab.* 2015 Aug;100(8):2918–26.

28 Jeon B, Baek J. Menstrual disturbances and its association with sleep disturbances: a systematic review. *BMC Womens Health.* 2023 Sep 1;23:470.

29 Baker FC, Lee KA. Menstrual Cycle Effects on Sleep. *Sleep Med Clin.* 2018 Sep;13(3):283–94.

30 Jehan S, Auguste E, Hussain M, Pandi-Perumal SR, Brzezinski A, Gupta R, et al. Sleep and Premenstrual Syndrome. *J Sleep Med Disord.* 2016;3(5):1061.

31 Moderie C, Boudreau P, Shechter A, Lespérance P, Boivin DB. Effects of exogenous melatonin on sleep and circadian rhythms in women with premenstrual dysphoric disorder. *Sleep.* 2021 Jul 8;44(12):zsab171.

32 Koikawa N, Takami Y, Kawasaki Y, Kawana F, Shiroshita N, Ogasawara E, et al. Changes in the objective measures of sleep between the initial nights of menses and the nights during the midfollicular phase of the menstrual cycle in collegiate female athletes. *Journal of Clinical Sleep Medicine.* 16(10):1745–51.

33 Jeong D, Lee H, Kim J. Effects of sleep pattern, duration, and quality on premenstrual syndrome and primary dysmenorrhea in korean high school girls. *BMC Women's Health.* 2023 Aug 28;23(1):456.

34 Kang W, Jang KH, Lim HM, Ahn JS, Park WJ. The menstrual cycle associated with insomnia in newly employed nurses performing shift

work: a 12-month follow-up study. *Int Arch Occup Environ Health.* 2019 Feb;92(2):227–35.

35 Kennedy KER, Onyeonwu C, Nowakowski S, Hale L, Branas CC, Killgore WDS, et al. Menstrual regularity and bleeding is associated with sleep duration, sleep quality and fatigue in a community sample. *J Sleep Res.* 2022 Feb;31(1):e13434.

36 Hu F, Wu C, Jia Y, Zhen H, Cheng H, Zhang F, et al. Shift work and menstruation: A meta-analysis study. *SSM – Population Health.* 2023 Dec 1;24:101542.

37 Lawson CC, Johnson CY, Chavarro JE, Lividoti Hibert EN, Whelan EA, Rocheleau CM, et al. Work schedule and physically demanding work in relation to menstrual function: the Nurses' Health Study 3. *Scandinavian Journal of Work, Environment & Health.* 2015;41(2):194–203.

38 Stocker LJ, Macklon NS, Cheong YC, Bewley SJ. Influence of shift work on early reproductive outcomes: a systematic review and meta-analysis. *Obstet Gynecol.* 2014 Jul;124(1):99–110.

39 Hu F, Wu C, Jia Y, Zhen H, Cheng H, Zhang F, et al. Shift work and menstruation: A meta-analysis study. *SSM – Population Health.* 2023 Dec 1;24:101542.

40 Lawson CC, Johnson CY, Chavarro JE, Lividoti Hibert EN, Whelan EA, Rocheleau CM, et al. Work schedule and physically demanding work in relation to menstrual function: the Nurses' Health Study 3. *Scandinavian Journal of Work, Environment & Health.* 2015;41(2):194–203.

41 Stocker LJ, Macklon NS, Cheong YC, Bewley SJ. Influence of shift work on early reproductive outcomes: a systematic review and meta-analysis. *Obstet Gynecol.* 2014 Jul;124(1):99–110.

42 Hu F, Wu C, Jia Y, Zhen H, Cheng H, Zhang F, et al. Shift work and menstruation: A meta-analysis study. *SSM – Population Health.* 2023 Dec 1;24:101542.

43 Stutz J, Eiholzer R, Spengler CM. Effects of Evening Exercise on Sleep in Healthy Participants: A Systematic Review and Meta-Analysis. *Sports Med.* 2019 Feb;49(2):269–87.

44 Bezerra AG, Andersen ML, Pires GN, Banzoli CV, Polesel DN, Tufik S, et al. Hormonal contraceptive use and subjective sleep reports in women: An online survey. *J Sleep Res.* 2020 Dec;29(6):e12983.

45 Bezerra AG, Andersen ML, Pires GN, Banzoli CV, Polesel DN, Tufik S, et al. Hormonal contraceptive use and subjective sleep reports in women: An online survey. *J Sleep Res*. 2020 Dec;29(6):e12983.

46 Hachul H, Andersen ML, Bittencourt L, Santos-Silva R, Tufik S. A population-based survey on the influence of the menstrual cycle and the use of hormonal contraceptives on sleep patterns in São Paulo, Brazil. *Int J Gynaecol Obstet*. 2013 Feb;120(2):137–40.

47 Hachul H, Andersen ML, Bittencourt LRA, Santos-Silva R, Conway SG, Tufik S. Does the reproductive cycle influence sleep patterns in women with sleep complaints? *Climacteric*. 2010 Dec;13(6):594–603.

48 Baker FC, Mitchell D, Driver HS. Oral contraceptives alter sleep and raise body temperature in young women. *Pflugers Arch*. 2001 Aug;442(5):729–37.

49 Plamberger CP, Van Wijk HE, Kerschbaum H, Pletzer BA, Gruber G, Oberascher K, et al. Impact of menstrual cycle phase and oral contraceptives on sleep and overnight memory consolidation. *J Sleep Res*. 2021 Aug;30(4):e13239.

50 Burdick RS, Hoffmann R, Armitage R. Short note: oral contraceptives and sleep in depressed and healthy women. *Sleep*. 2002 May 1;25(3):347–9.

51 Institute of Medicine (US) Committee on Military NutritionInstitute of Medicine (US) Committee on Military NutritionInstitute of Medicine (US) Committee on Military Nutrition. Pharmacology of Caffeine. In: Caffeine for the Sustainment of Mental Task Performance: Formulations for Military Operations. National Academies Press (US); 2001.

Mood

1 Kuehner C. Why is depression more common among women than among men? *Lancet Psychiatry*. 2017 Feb;4(2):146–58.

2 Freeman EW. Associations of depression with the transition to menopause. *Menopause*. 2010 Jul;17(4):823.

3 Wieczorek K, Targonskaya A, Maslowski K. Reproductive Hormones and Female Mental Wellbeing. *Women*. 2023 Sep;3(3):432–44.

4 Del Río JP, Alliende MI, Molina N, Serrano FG, Molina S, Vigil P. Steroid Hormones and Their Action in Women's Brains: The Importance of Hormonal Balance. *Front Public Health* 2018 May 23;6.

5 Wieczorek K, Targonskaya A, Maslowski K. Reproductive Hormones and Female Mental Wellbeing. *Women*. 2023 Sep;3(3):432–44.

6 Del Río JP, Alliende MI, Molina N, Serrano FG, Molina S, Vigil P. Steroid Hormones and Their Action in Women's Brains: The Importance of Hormonal Balance. *Front Public Health* 2018 May 23;6.

7 Sundström-Poromaa I, Comasco E, Sumner R, Luders E. Progesterone – Friend or foe? *Front Neuroendocrinol.* 2020 Oct;59:100856.

8 Bixo M, Johansson M, Timby E, Michalski L, Bäckström T. Effects of GABA active steroids in the female brain with a focus on the premenstrual dysphoric disorder. *J Neuroendocrinol.* 2018 Feb;30(2).

9 Bäckström T, Bixo M, Johansson M, Nyberg S, Ossewaarde L, Ragagnin G, et al. Allopregnanolone and mood disorders. *Prog Neurobiol.* 2014 Feb;113:88–94.

10 Cyranowski JM, Frank E, Young E, Shear MK. Adolescent onset of the gender difference in lifetime rates of major depression: a theoretical model. *Arch Gen Psychiatry.* 2000 Jan;57(1):21–7.

11 Angold A, Worthman CW. Puberty onset of gender differences in rates of depression: a developmental, epidemiologic and neuroendocrine perspective. *J Affect Disord.* 1993;29(2–3):145–58.

12 Oliver KK, Thelen MH. Children's perceptions of peer influence on eating concerns. *Behavior Therapy.* 1996 Dec 1;27(1):25–39.

13 Lawler M, Nixon E. Body dissatisfaction among adolescent boys and girls: the effects of body mass, peer appearance culture and internalization of appearance ideals. *J Youth Adolesc.* 2011 Jan;40(1):59–71.

14 Herrmann J, Koeppen K, Kessels U. Do girls take school too seriously? Investigating gender differences in school burnout from a self-worth perspective. *Learning and Individual Differences.* 2019 Jan 1;69:150–61.

15 Martell S, Marini C, Kondas CA, Deutch AB. Psychological side effects of hormonal contraception: a disconnect between patients and providers. *Contracept Reprod Med.* 2023 Jan 17;8:9.

16 Martell S, Marini C, Kondas CA, Deutch AB. Psychological side effects of hormonal contraception: a disconnect between patients and providers. *Contracept Reprod Med.* 2023 Jan 17;8:9.

17 Herzberg BN, Draper KC, Johnson AL, Nicol GC. Oral Contraceptives, Depression, and Libido. *Br Med J.* 1971 Aug 28;3(5773):495–500.

18 Skovlund CW, Mørch LS, Kessing LV, Lidegaard Ø. Association of Hormonal Contraception With Depression. *JAMA Psychiatry.* 2016 Nov 1;73(11):1154–62.

19 Zethraeus N, Dreber A, Ranehill E, Blomberg L, Labrie F, von Schoultz B, et al. A first-choice combined oral contraceptive influences general well-being in healthy women: a double-blind, randomized, placebo-controlled trial. *Fertil Steril.* 2017 May;107(5):1238–45.

20 Toffol E, Heikinheimo O, Koponen P, Luoto R, Partonen T. Hormonal contraception and mental health: results of a population-based study. *Hum Reprod.* 2011 Nov;26(11):3085–93.

21 Keyes KM, Cheslack-Postava K, Westhoff C, Heim CM, Haloossim M, Walsh K, et al. Association of hormonal contraceptive use with reduced levels of depressive symptoms: a national study of sexually active women in the United States. *Am J Epidemiol.* 2013 Nov 1;178(9):1378–88.

22 Svendal G, Berk M, Pasco JA, Jacka FN, Lund A, Williams LJ. The use of hormonal contraceptive agents and mood disorders in women. *J Affect Disord.* 2012 Sep;140(1):92–6.

23 Mu E, Kulkarni J. Hormonal contraception and mood disorders. *Aust Prescr.* 2022 Jun;45(3):75–9.

24 Schaffir J, Worly BL, Gur TL. Combined hormonal contraception and its effects on mood: a critical review. *Eur J Contracept Reprod Health Care.* 2016 Oct;21(5):347–55.

25 Schaffir J, Worly BL, Gur TL. Combined hormonal contraception and its effects on mood: a critical review. *Eur J Contracept Reprod Health Care.* 2016 Oct;21(5):347–55.

26 Schoep ME, Nieboer TE, van der Zanden M, Braat DDM, Nap AW. The impact of menstrual symptoms on everyday life: a survey among 42,879 women. *Am J Obstet Gynecol.* 2019 Jun;220(6):569.e1-569.e7.

27 NICE Guideline. Premenstrual syndrome | CKS | NICE [Internet]. [cited 2024 Jun 18]. Available from: https://cks.nice.org.uk/topics/premenstrual-syndrome/

28 Gao M, Zhang H, Gao Z, Cheng X, Sun Y, Qiao M, et al. Global and regional prevalence and burden for premenstrual syndrome and premenstrual dysphoric disorder. *Medicine* (Baltimore). 2022 Jan 7;101(1):e28528.

29 Halbreich U, Borenstein J, Pearlstein T, Kahn LS. The prevalence, impairment, impact, and burden of premenstrual dysphoric disorder (PMS/PMDD). *Psychoneuroendocrinology.* 2003 Aug;28 Suppl 3:1–23.

30 Halbreich U, Borenstein J, Pearlstein T, Kahn LS. The prevalence, impairment, impact, and burden of premenstrual dysphoric disorder (PMS/PMDD). *Psychoneuroendocrinology.* 2003 Aug;28 Suppl 3:1–23.

31 Hantsoo L, Epperson CN. Premenstrual Dysphoric Disorder: Epidemi-
    ology and Treatment. *Curr Psychiatry Rep.* 2015 Nov;17(11):87.

32 Hantsoo L, Epperson CN. Allopregnanolone in premenstrual dysphoric
    disorder (PMDD): Evidence for dysregulated sensitivity to GABA-A
    receptor modulating neuroactive steroids across the menstrual cycle.
    Neurobiol Stress. 2020 Feb 4;12:100213.

33 Hantsoo L, Payne JL. Towards understanding the biology of premenstrual
    dysphoric disorder: From genes to GABA. *Neuroscience & Biobehavioral
    Reviews.* 2023 Jun 1;149:105168.

34 Wilson CA, Turner CW, Keye WR. Firstborn adolescent daughters and
    mothers with and without premenstrual syndrome: A comparison. *Jour-
    nal of Adolescent Health.* 1991 Mar 1;12(2):130–7.

35 Kendler KS, Silberg JL, Neale MC, Kessler RC, Heath AC, Eaves LJ.
    Genetic and environmental factors in the aetiology of menstrual, pre-
    menstrual and neurotic symptoms: a population-based twin study.
    Psychol Med. 1992 Feb;22(1):85–100.

36 IAPMD [Internet]. [cited 2024 Jun 18]. What is PME. Available from:
    https://iapmd.org/pmdd-v-pme

37 Osborn E, Wittkowski A, Brooks J, Briggs PE, O'Brien PMS. Women's
    experiences of receiving a diagnosis of premenstrual dysphoric dis-
    order: a qualitative investigation. *BMC Women's Health.* 2020 Oct
    28;20(1):242.

38 Osborn E, Wittkowski A, Brooks J, Briggs PE, O'Brien PMS. Women's
    experiences of receiving a diagnosis of premenstrual dysphoric disorder:
    a qualitative investigation. *BMC Women's Health.* 2020 Oct 28;20(1):242.

39 McManus S, Bebbington PE, Jenkins R, Brugha T. Mental Health and
    Wellbeing in England: the Adult Psychiatric Morbidity Survey 2014
    [Internet]. Leeds, UK: NHS Digital; 2016 [cited 2024 Jun 18].

40 Siminiuc R, Țurcanu D. Impact of nutritional diet therapy on premen-
    strual syndrome. *Front Nutr.* 2023 Feb 1;10:1079417.

41 Houghton SC, Manson JE, Whitcomb BW, Hankinson SE, Troy LM,
    Bigelow C, et al. Carbohydrate and fiber intake and the risk of premen-
    strual syndrome. *Eur J Clin Nutr.* 2018 Jun;72(6):861–70.

42 van Die MD, Burger HG, Teede HJ, Bone KM. Vitex agnus-castus
    extracts for female reproductive disorders: a systematic review of clinical
    trials. *Planta Med.* 2013 May;79(7):562–75.

43 Verkaik S, Kamperman AM, van Westrhenen R, Schulte PFJ. The treatment of premenstrual syndrome with preparations of Vitex agnus castus: a systematic review and meta-analysis. *Am J Obstet Gynecol.* 2017 Aug;217(2):150–66.

44 Cerqueira RO, Frey BN, Leclerc E, Brietzke E. Vitex agnus castus for premenstrual syndrome and premenstrual dysphoric disorder: a systematic review. *Arch Womens Ment Health.* 2017 Dec;20(6):713–9.

45 Thys-Jacobs S, Ceccarelli S, Bierman A, Weisman H, Cohen MA, Alvir J. Calcium supplementation in premenstrual syndrome: a randomized crossover trial. *J Gen Intern Med.* 1989;4(3):183–9.

46 Thys-Jacobs S, Starkey P, Bernstein D, Tian J. Calcium carbonate and the premenstrual syndrome: effects on premenstrual and menstrual symptoms. Premenstrual Syndrome Study Group. *Am J Obstet Gynecol.* 1998 Aug;179(2):444–52.

47 Yonkers KA, Pearlstein TB, Gotman N. A pilot study to compare fluoxetine, calcium, and placebo in the treatment of premenstrual syndrome. *J Clin Psychopharmacol.* 2013 Oct;33(5):614–20.

48 Bertone-Johnson ER, Hankinson SE, Bendich A, Johnson SR, Willett WC, Manson JE. Calcium and vitamin D intake and risk of incident premenstrual syndrome. *Arch Intern Med.* 2005 Jun 13;165(11):1246–52.

49 Abdi F, Ozgoli G, Rahnemaie FS. A systematic review of the role of vitamin D and calcium in premenstrual syndrome. *Obstet Gynecol Sci.* 2019 Mar;62(2):73–86.

50 Walker AF, De Souza MC, Vickers MF, Abeyasekera S, Collins ML, Trinca LA. Magnesium supplementation alleviates premenstrual symptoms of fluid retention. *J Womens Health.* 1998 Nov;7(9):1157–65.

51 Quaranta S, Buscaglia MA, Meroni MG, Colombo E, Cella S. Pilot study of the efficacy and safety of a modified-release magnesium 250 mg tablet (Sincromag) for the treatment of premenstrual syndrome. *Clin Drug Investig.* 2007;27(1):51–8.

52 Facchinetti F, Borella P, Sances G, Fioroni L, Nappi RE, Genazzani AR. Oral magnesium successfully relieves premenstrual mood changes. *Obstet Gynecol.* 1991 Aug;78(2):177–81.

53 Fathizadeh N, Ebrahimi E, Valiani M, Tavakoli N, Yar MH. Evaluating the effect of magnesium and magnesium plus vitamin B6 supplement on the severity of premenstrual syndrome. *Iran J Nurs Midwifery Res.* 2010 Dec;15(Suppl1):401–5.

54 Wyatt KM, Dimmock PW, Jones PW, Shaughn O'Brien PM. Efficacy of vitamin B-6 in the treatment of premenstrual syndrome: systematic review. *BMJ*. 1999 May 22;318(7195):1375–81.

55 Pearce E, Jolly K, Jones LL, Matthewman G, Zanganeh M, Daley A. Exercise for premenstrual syndrome: a systematic review and meta-analysis of randomised controlled trials. *BJGP Open*. 4(3):bjgpopen20X101032.

56 Ma S, Song SJ. Oral contraceptives containing drospirenone for premenstrual syndrome – Ma, S – 2023 | Cochrane Library.

57 RCOG . Managing premenstrual syndrome (PMS). Available from: https://www.rcog.org.uk/for-the-public/browse-our-patient-information/managing-premenstrual-syndrome-pms/

58 Hunter MS, Ussher JM, Browne SJ, Cariss M, Jelley R, Katz M. A randomized comparison of psychological (cognitive behavior therapy), medical (fluoxetine) and combined treatment for women with premenstrual dysphoric disorder. *J Psychosom Obstet Gynaecol*. 2002 Sep;23(3):193–9.

Breast health

1 Love SM, Lindsey K, Love E. *Dr. Susan Love's Breast Book*. Hachette Books; 2015. (A Merloyd Lawrence Book).

2 Breast asymmetry: Women in Dorset share their experiences. BBC News [Internet]. 2023 Jun 13 [cited 2024 Jun 17]; Available from: https://www.bbc.com/news/uk-england-dorset-65883917

3 Ramakrishnan R, Khan SA, Badve S. Morphological Changes in Breast Tissue with Menstrual Cycle. *Mod Pathol*. 2002 Dec;15(12):1348–56.

4 Wang C, Luan J, Cheng H, Chen L, Li Z, Panayi AC, et al. Menstrual Cycle-Related Fluctuations in Breast Volume Measured Using Three-Dimensional Imaging: Implications for Volumetric Evaluation in Breast Augmentation. *Aesthetic Plast Surg*. 2019 Feb;43(1):1–6.

5 Fowler PA, Casey CE, Cameron GG, Foster MA, Knight CH. Cyclic changes in composition and volume of the breast during the menstrual cycle, measured by magnetic resonance imaging. *Br J Obstet Gynaecol*. 1990 Jul;97(7):595–602.

6 Ramakrishnan R, Khan SA, Badve S. Morphological Changes in Breast Tissue with Menstrual Cycle. *Mod Pathol*. 2002 Dec;15(12):1348–56.

7 Fowler PA, Casey CE, Cameron GG, Foster MA, Knight CH. Cyclic changes in composition and volume of the breast during the menstrual

cycle, measured by magnetic resonance imaging. *Br J Obstet Gynaecol.* 1990 Jul;97(7):595–602.

8 Hussain Z, Roberts N, Whitehouse GH, García-Fiñana M, Percy D. Estimation of breast volume and its variation during the menstrual cycle using MRI and stereology. *British Journal of Radiology.* 1999 Mar 1;72(855):236–45.

9 The Pill and Boobs [Internet]. The Lowdown. 2022 [cited 2024 Jun 17]. Available from: https://thelowdown.com/blog/the-pill-and-boobs

10 Lopez LM, Grimes DA, Gallo MF, Stockton LL, Schulz KF. Skin patch and vaginal ring versus combined oral contraceptives for contraception – Lopez, LM – 2013 | Cochrane Library. [cited 2024 Jun 17]; Available from: https://www.cochranelibrary.com/cdsr/doi/10.1002/14651858.CD0035 52.pub4/full

11 Luukkainen T, Pakarinen P, Toivonen J. Progestin-Releasing Intrauterine Systems. *Seminars in Reproductive Medicine.* 2001 Nov 29;19:355–64.

12 Hunt JT, Kamat R, Yao M, Sharma N, Batur P. Effect of contraceptive hormonal therapy on mammographic breast density: A longitudinal cohort study. *Clinical Imaging.* 2023 May 1;97:62–7.

13 NICE Guideline. Breast pain – cyclical | CKS | NICE.

14 Ader DN, Browne MW. Prevalence and impact of cyclic mastalgia in a United States clinic-based sample. *American Journal of Obstetrics & Gynecology.* 1997 Jul 1;177(1):126–32.

15 Goyal A. Breast pain. *BMJ Clin Evid.* 2011 Jan 17;2011:0812.

16 NICE Guideline. Breast pain – cyclical | CKS | NICE.

17 Goyal A. Breast pain. *BMJ Clin Evid.* 2011 Jan 17;2011:0812.

18 Ahmad Adni LL, Norhayati MN, Mohd Rosli RR, Muhammad J. A Systematic Review and Meta-Analysis of the Efficacy of Evening Primrose Oil for Mastalgia Treatment. *Int J Environ Res Public Health.* 2021 Jun 10;18(12):6295.

19 Pruthi S, Wahner-Roedler DL, Torkelson CJ, Cha SS, Thicke LS, Hazelton JH, et al. Vitamin E and evening primrose oil for management of cyclical mastalgia: a randomized pilot study. *Altern Med Rev.* 2010 Apr;15(1):59–67.

20 Ooi SL, Watts S, McClean R, Pak SC. Vitex Agnus-Castus for the Treatment of Cyclic Mastalgia: A Systematic Review and Meta-Analysis. *J Womens Health* (Larchmt). 2020 Feb;29(2):262–78.

21 Mirghafourvand M, Mohammad-Alizadeh-Charandabi S, Ahmadpour P, Javadzadeh Y. Effects of Vitex agnus and Flaxseed on cyclic mastalgia: A randomized controlled trial. *Complement Ther Med.* 2016 Feb;24:90–5.

22 European Union herbal monograph on Vitex agnus-castus L., fructus.

23 Jaafarnejad F, Adibmoghaddam E, Emami SA, Saki A. Compare the effect of flaxseed, evening primrose oil and Vitamin E on duration of periodic breast pain. *J Educ Health Promot.* 2017;6:85.

24 Godazandeh G, Ala S, Motlaq TM, Sahebnasagh A, Bazi A. The comparison of the effect of flaxseed oil and vitamin E on mastalgia and nodularity of breast fibrocystic: a randomized double-blind clinical trial. *Journal of Pharmaceutical Health Care and Sciences.* 2021 Jan 6;7(1):4.

25 Gehlsen G, Albohm M. Evaluation of Sports Bras. *Phys Sportsmed.* 1980 Oct;8(10):88–97.

26 Brown N, Burnett E, Scurr J. Is Breast Pain Greater in Active Females Compared to the General Population in the UK? *Breast J.* 2016;22(2):194–201.

27 Gehlsen G, Albohm M. Evaluation of Sports Bras. *Phys Sportsmed.* 1980 Oct;8(10):88–97.

28 Bridgman C, Scurr J, White J, Hedger W, Galbraith H. Three-dimensional kinematics of the breast during a two-step star jump. *J Appl Biomech.* 2010 Nov;26(4):465–72.

29 Scurr JC, White JL, Hedger W. Supported and unsupported breast displacement in three dimensions across treadmill activity levels. *J Sports Sci.* 2011 Jan;29(1):55–61.

30 Mason BR, Page KA, Fallon K. An analysis of movement and discomfort of the female breast during exercise and the effects of breast support in three cases. *J Sci Med Sport.* 1999 Jun;2(2):134–44.

31 McGhee DE, Steele JR. Biomechanics of Breast Support for Active Women. *Exerc Sport Sci Rev.* 2020 Jul;48(3):99–109.

32 Burnett E, White J, Scurr J. The Influence of the Breast on Physical Activity Participation in Females. *J Phys Act Health.* 2015 Apr;12(4):588–94.

33 Burnett E, White J, Scurr J. The Influence of the Breast on Physical Activity Participation in Females. *J Phys Act Health.* 2015 Apr;12(4):588–94.

34 Routledge & CRC Press [Internet]. [cited 2024 Jun 17]. The Exercising Female: Science and Its Application. Available from: https://www.routledge.com/The-Exercising-Female-Science-and-Its-Application/Forsyth-Roberts/p/book/9780367615925

35 Brown N, Scurr J. Do women with smaller breasts perform better in long-distance running? *Eur J Sport Sci.* 2016 Nov;16(8):965–71.

36 Milligan A, Mills C, Corbett J, Scurr J. The influence of breast support on torso, pelvis and arm kinematics during a five kilometer treadmill run. *Hum Mov Sci.* 2015 Aug;42:246–60.

37 Breastcancer.org, Uscher J, Santora T. Breast self-exam guidelines. Breast Self-Exam. Available from: https://www.breastcancer.org/screening-test ing/breast-self-exam-bse

Body image

1 Papathomas A, White HJ, Plateau CR. Young people, social media, and disordered eating. In: *Young People, Social Media and Health.* Routledge; 2018.

2 Bornioli A, Lewis-Smith H, Slater A, Bray I. Body dissatisfaction predicts the onset of depression among adolescent females and males: a prospective study. *J Epidemiol Community Health.* 2021 Apr 1;75(4):343–8.

3 Bauer A, Schneider S, Waldorf M, Adolph D, Vocks S. Familial transmission of a body-related attentional bias – An eye-tracking study in a nonclinical sample of female adolescents and their mothers. *PLoS One.* 2017 Nov 27;12(11):e0188186.

4 Keery H, van den Berg P, Thompson JK. An evaluation of the Tripartite Influence Model of body dissatisfaction and eating disturbance with adolescent girls. *Body Image.* 2004 Sep;1(3):237–51.

5 Kluck AS. Family influence on disordered eating: the role of body image dissatisfaction. *Body Image.* 2010 Jan;7(1):8–14.

6 Rodgers RF, Paxton SJ, Chabrol H. Effects of parental comments on body dissatisfaction and eating disturbance in young adults: a sociocultural model. *Body Image.* 2009 Jun;6(3):171–7.

7 Schwartz DJ, Phares V, Tantleff-Dunn S, Thompson JK. Body image, psychological functioning, and parental feedback regarding physical appearance. *International Journal of Eating Disorders.* 1999;25(3):339–43.

8 Carbonneau N, Goodman LC, Roberts LT, Bégin C, Lussier Y, Musher-Eizenman DR. A look at the intergenerational associations between self-compassion, body esteem, and emotional eating within dyads of mothers and their adult daughters. *Body Image.* 2020 Jun;33:106–14.

9 Tompkins KB, Martz DM, Rocheleau CA, Bazzini DG. Social likeability,

conformity, and body talk: Does fat talk have a normative rival in female body image conversations? *Body Image*. 2009 Sep 1;6(4):292–8.

10 Rusticus S. Body Image. In: Michalos A C, editor. *Encyclopedia of Quality of Life and Well-Being Research* [Internet]. Dordrecht: Springer Netherlands; 2014 [cited 2024 Jun 17]. p. 420–3. Available from: https://doi.org/10.1007/978-94-007-0753-5_224

11 Krohmer K, Derntl B, Svaldi J. Hormones Matter? Association of the Menstrual Cycle With Selective Attention for Liked and Disliked Body Parts. *Front Psychol*. 2019 May 8;10:851.

12 Durante K M, Li N P, Haselton M G. Changes in women's choice of dress across the ovulatory cycle: naturalistic and laboratory task-based evidence. *Pers Soc Psychol Bull*. 2008 Nov;34(11):1451–60.

13 Haselton M G, Gangestad S W. Conditional expression of women's desires and men's mate guarding across the ovulatory cycle. *Horm Behav*. 2006 Apr;49(4):509–18.

14 Durante K M, Li N P, Haselton M G. Changes in women's choice of dress across the ovulatory cycle: naturalistic and laboratory task-based evidence. *Pers Soc Psychol Bull*. 2008 Nov;34(11):1451–60.

15 Krohmer K, Derntl B, Svaldi J. Hormones Matter? Association of the Menstrual Cycle With Selective Attention for Liked and Disliked Body Parts. *Front Psychol*. 2019 May 8;10:851.

16 Teixeira A L S, Dias M R C, Damasceno V O, Lamounier J A, Gardner R M. Association between different phases of menstrual cycle and body image measures of perceived size, ideal size, and body dissatisfaction. *Percept Mot Skills*. 2013 Dec;117(3):892–902.

17 Kanellakis S, Skoufas E, Simitsopoulou E, Migdanis A, Migdanis I, Prelorentzou T, et al. Changes in body weight and body composition during the menstrual cycle. *American Journal of Human Biology*. 2023;35(11):e23951.

18 White C P, Hitchcock C L, Vigna Y M, Prior J C. Fluid Retention over the Menstrual Cycle: 1-Year Data from the Prospective Ovulation Cohort. *Obstet Gynecol Int*. 2011;2011:138451.

19 Ussher J M, Perz J. Evaluation of the relative efficacy of a couple cognitive-behaviour therapy (C B T) for Premenstrual Disorders (P M D s), in comparison to one-to-one C B T and a wait list control: A randomized controlled trial. *PL oS One*. 2017 Apr 18;12(4):e0175068.

20 Ussher JM, Perz J. Evaluation of the relative efficacy of a couple cognitive-behaviour therapy (CBT) for Premenstrual Disorders (PMDs), in comparison to one-to-one CBT and a wait list control: A randomized controlled trial. *PLoS One.* 2017 Apr 18;12(4):e0175068.

21 Ryan S, Ussher JM, Hawkey A. Managing the premenstrual body: a body mapping study of women's negotiation of premenstrual food cravings and exercise. *Journal of Eating Disorders.* 2021 Oct 9;9(1):125.

22 Chrisler JC, Marván ML, Gorman JA, Rossini M. Body appreciation and attitudes toward menstruation. *Body Image.* 2015 Jan;12:78–81.

23 Krohmer K, Derntl B, Svaldi J. Hormones Matter? Association of the Menstrual Cycle With Selective Attention for Liked and Disliked Body Parts. *Front Psychol.* 2019 May 8;10:851.

24 Bird JL, Oinonen KA. Elevated eating disorder symptoms in women with a history of oral contraceptive side effects. *Arch Womens Ment Health.* 2011 Aug 1;14(4):345–53.

25 Gallo MF, Lopez LM, Grimes DA, Carayon F, Schulz KF, Helmerhorst FM. Combination contraceptives: effects on weight – Gallo, MF – 2014 | Cochrane Library. [cited 2024 Jun 17]; Available from: https://www.cochranelibrary.com/cdsr/doi/10.1002/14651858.CD003987.pub5/full

26 Gillen MM. Associations between positive body image and indicators of men's and women's mental and physical health. *Body Image.* 2015 Mar 1;13:67–74.

27 Homan KJ, Tylka TL. Appearance-based exercise motivation moderates the relationship between exercise frequency and positive body image. *Body Image.* 2014 Mar;11(2):101–8.

28 Homan KJ, Tylka TL. Appearance-based exercise motivation moderates the relationship between exercise frequency and positive body image. *Body Image.* 2014 Mar;11(2):101–8.

29 Gilchrist JD, Pila E, Castonguay A, Sabiston CM, Mack DE. Body pride and physical activity: Differential associations between fitness- and appearance-related pride in young adult Canadians. *Body Image.* 2018 Dec;27:77–85.

30 Jiotsa B, Naccache B, Duval M, Rocher B, Grall-Bronnec M. Social Media Use and Body Image Disorders: Association between Frequency of Comparing One's Own Physical Appearance to That of People Being Followed on Social Media and Body Dissatisfaction and Drive for Thinness. *Int J Environ Res Public Health.* 2021 Mar 11;18(6):2880.

31 Cataldo I, De Luca I, Giorgetti V, Cicconcelli D, Bersani F S, Imperatori C, et al. Fitspiration on social media: Body-image and other psychopathological risks among young adults. A narrative review. *Emerging Trends in Drugs, Addictions, and Health*. 2021 Jan 1;1:100010.

32 Jerónimo F, Carraça E V. Effects of fitspiration content on body image: a systematic review. *Eat Weight Disord*. 2022 Dec;27(8):3017–35.

Sex and libido

1 Eftekhar T, Sohrabvand F, Zabandan N, Shariat M, Haghollahi F, Ghahghaei-Nezamabadi A. Sexual dysfunction in patients with polycystic ovary syndrome and its affected domains. *Iran J Reprod Med*. 2014 Aug;12(8):539–46.

2 Roney J R, Simmons Z L. Hormonal predictors of sexual motivation in natural menstrual cycles. *Hormones and Behavior*. 2013 Apr 1;63(4): 636–45.

3 Roney J R, Simmons Z L. Hormonal predictors of sexual motivation in natural menstrual cycles. *Hormones and Behavior*. 2013 Apr 1;63(4):636–45.

4 Van Goozen S H, Wiegant V M, Endert E, Helmond F A, Van de Poll N E. Psychoendocrinological assessment of the menstrual cycle: the relationship between hormones, sexuality, and mood. *Arch Sex Behav*. 1997 Aug;26(4):359–82.

5 Kiesner J, Bittoni C, Eisenlohr-Moul T, Komisaruk B, Pastore M. Menstrual cycle-driven vs noncyclical daily changes in sexual desire. *J Sex Med*. 2023 May 26;20(6):756–65.

6 Pastor Z, Holla K, Chmel R. The influence of combined oral contraceptives on female sexual desire: a systematic review. *Eur J Contracept Reprod Health Care*. 2013 Feb 1;18(1):27–43.

7 Pastor Z, Holla K, Chmel R. The influence of combined oral contraceptives on female sexual desire: a systematic review. *Eur J Contracept Reprod Health Care*. 2013 Feb 1;18(1):27–43.

8 Zethraeus N, Dreber A, Ranehill E, Blomberg L, Labrie F, von Schoultz B, et al. Combined Oral Contraceptives and Sexual Function in Women-a Double-Blind, Randomized, Placebo-Controlled Trial. *J Clin Endocrinol Metab*. 2016 Nov;101(11):4046–53.

9 Zethraeus N, Dreber A, Ranehill E, Blomberg L, Labrie F, von Schoultz B, et al. Combined Oral Contraceptives and Sexual Function in Women-a

Double-Blind, Randomized, Placebo-Controlled Trial. *J Clin Endocrinol Metab.* 2016 Nov;101(11):4046–53.

10 Zethraeus N, Dreber A, Ranehill E, Blomberg L, Labrie F, von Schoultz B, et al. Combined Oral Contraceptives and Sexual Function in Women-a Double-Blind, Randomized, Placebo-Controlled Trial. *J Clin Endocrinol Metab.* 2016 Nov;101(11):4046–53.

11 Sanders SA, Graham CA, Bass JL, Bancroft J. A prospective study of the effects of oral contraceptives on sexuality and well-being and their relationship to discontinuation. *Contraception.* 2001 Jul;64(1):51–8.

12 #menstrubation [Internet]. [cited 2024 Jun 18]. Menstrubation: can masturbation help with menstruation pain? Available from: https://menstrubation.com/

Skin and hair

1 Geller L, Rosen J, Frankel A, Goldenberg G. Perimenstrual Flare of Adult Acne. *J Clin Aesthet Dermatol.* 2014 Aug;7(8):30–4.

2 Raghunath RS, Venables ZC, Millington GWM. The menstrual cycle and the skin. *Clin Exp Dermatol.* 2015 Mar;40(2):111–5.

3 Raghunath RS, Venables ZC, Millington GWM. The menstrual cycle and the skin. *Clin Exp Dermatol.* 2015 Mar;40(2):111–5.

4 Gratton R, Del Vecchio C, Zupin L, Crovella S. Unraveling the Role of Sex Hormones on Keratinocyte Functions in Human Inflammatory Skin Diseases. *Int J Mol Sci.* 2022 Mar 15;23(6):3132.

5 Jacobsen E, Billings JK, Frantz RA, Kinney CK, Stewart ME, Downing DT. Age-related changes in sebaceous wax ester secretion rates in men and women. *J Invest Dermatol.* 1985 Nov;85(5):483–5.

6 Shah MG, Maibach HI. Estrogen and skin. An overview. *Am J Clin Dermatol.* 2001;2(3):143–50.

7 Grymowicz M, Rudnicka E, Podfigurna A, Napierala P, Smolarczyk R, Smolarczyk K, et al. *Hormonal Effects on Hair Follicles.* Int J Mol Sci. 2020 Jul 28;21(15):5342.

8 Shah MG, Maibach HI. Estrogen and skin. An overview. *Am J Clin Dermatol.* 2001;2(3):143–50.

9 Gratton R, Del Vecchio C, Zupin L, Crovella S. Unraveling the Role of Sex Hormones on Keratinocyte Functions in Human Inflammatory Skin Diseases. *Int J Mol Sci.* 2022 Mar 15;23(6):3132.

10 Elsaie ML. Hormonal treatment of acne vulgaris: an update. *Clin Cosmet Investig Dermatol.* 2016 Sep 2;9:241–8.

11 Wright PJ, CORBETT CF, PINTO BM, DAWSON RM, WIRTH M. Resistance Training as Therapeutic Management in Women with PCOS: What is the Evidence? *Int J Exerc Sci.* 2021 Aug 1;14(3):840–54.

12 Cutler DA, Pride SM, Cheung AP. Low intakes of dietary fiber and magnesium are associated with insulin resistance and hyperandrogenism in polycystic ovary syndrome: A cohort study. *Food Sci Nutr.* 2019 Apr;7(4):1426–37.

13 Sørensen LB, Søe M, Halkier KH, Stigsby B, Astrup A. Effects of increased dietary protein-to-carbohydrate ratios in women with polycystic ovary syndrome. *Am J Clin Nutr.* 2012 Jan;95(1):39–48.

14 Shah MG, Maibach HI. Estrogen and skin. An overview. *Am J Clin Dermatol.* 2001;2(3):143–50.

15 Agner T, Damm P, Skouby SO. Menstrual cycle and skin reactivity. *J Am Acad Dermatol.* 1991 Apr;24(4):566–70.

16 Shah MG, Maibach HI. Estrogen and skin. An overview. *Am J Clin Dermatol.* 2001;2(3):143–50.

17 Raghunath RS, Venables ZC, Millington GWM. The menstrual cycle and the skin. *Clin Exp Dermatol.* 2015 Mar;40(2):111–5.

18 Cario M. How hormones may modulate human skin pigmentation in melasma: An in vitro perspective. *Exp Dermatol.* 2019 Jun;28(6):709–18.

19 Cario M. How hormones may modulate human skin pigmentation in melasma: An in vitro perspective. *Exp Dermatol.* 2019 Jun;28(6):709–18.

20 Raghunath RS, Venables ZC, Millington GWM. The menstrual cycle and the skin. *Clin Exp Dermatol.* 2015 Mar;40(2):111–5.

21 Geller L, Rosen J, Frankel A, Goldenberg G. Perimenstrual Flare of Adult Acne. *J Clin Aesthet Dermatol.* 2014 Aug;7(8):30–4.

22 Dai R, Hua W, Chen W, Xiong L, Li L. The effect of milk consumption on acne: a meta-analysis of observational studies. *J Eur Acad Dermatol Venereol.* 2018 Dec;32(12):2244–53.

23 Baldwin H, Tan J. Effects of Diet on Acne and Its Response to Treatment. *Am J Clin Dermatol.* 2021 Jan;22(1):55–65.

24 Dai R, Hua W, Chen W, Xiong L, Li L. The effect of milk consumption on acne: a meta-analysis of observational studies. *J Eur Acad Dermatol Venereol.* 2018 Dec;32(12):2244–53.

25 Baldwin H, Tan J. Effects of Diet on Acne and Its Response to Treatment. *Am J Clin Dermatol.* 2021 Jan;22(1):55–65.

26 Baldwin H, Tan J. Effects of Diet on Acne and Its Response to Treatment. *Am J Clin Dermatol.* 2021 Jan;22(1):55–65.

27 Burris J, Shikany J M, Rietkerk W, Woolf K. A Low Glycemic Index and Glycemic Load Diet Decreases Insulin-like Growth Factor-1 among Adults with Moderate and Severe Acne: A Short-Duration, 2-Week Randomized Controlled Trial. *J Acad Nutr Diet.* 2018 Oct;118(10):1874–85.

28 Pavithra G, Upadya G M, Rukmini M S. A randomized controlled trial of topical benzoyl peroxide 2.5% gel with a low glycemic load diet versus topical benzoyl peroxide 2.5% gel with a normal diet in acne (grades 1-3). *Indian J Dermatol Venereol Leprol.* 2019;85(5):486–90.

29 Birch M P, Messenger A. 'Bad hair days', scalp sebum excretion and the menstrual cycle. *J Cosmet Dermatol.* 2003 Jul;2(3–4):190–4.

30 Munro M G. Heavy menstrual bleeding, iron deficiency, and iron deficiency anemia: Framing the issue. *International Journal of Gynecology & Obstetrics.* 2023;162(S2):7–13.

31 nhs.uk [Internet]. 2017 [cited 2024 Jun 18]. Iron deficiency anaemia. Available from: https://www.nhs.uk/conditions/iron-deficiency-anaemia/

32 van Zuuren E J, Fedorowicz Z, Carter B, Pandis N. Interventions for hirsutism (excluding laser and photoepilation therapy alone). *Cochrane Database Syst Rev.* 2015 Apr 28;2015(4):CD010334.

33 Arowojolu A O, Gallo M F, Lopez L M, Grimes D A. Combined oral contraceptive pills for treatment of acne – Arowojolu, A O – 2012 | Cochrane Library. [cited 2024 Jun 18]; Available from: https://www.cochranelibrary.com/cdsr/doi/10.1002/14651858.CD004425.pub6/full

34 Williams N M, Randolph M, Rajabi-Estarabadi A, Keri J, Tosti A. Hormonal Contraceptives and Dermatology. *Am J Clin Dermatol.* 2021 Jan;22(1):69–80.

35 Raudrant D, Rabe T. Progestogens with antiandrogenic properties. *Drugs.* 2003;63(5):463–92.

36 Jones E E. Androgenic effects of oral contraceptives: implications for patient compliance. *Am J Med.* 1995 Jan 16;98(1A):116S-119S.

37 Barbieri J S, Mitra N, Margolis D J, Harper C C, Mostaghimi A, Abuabara K. Influence of Contraception Class on Incidence and Severity of Acne Vulgaris. *Obstet Gynecol.* 2020 Jun;135(6):1306–12.

Part 3: Getting Support

Speaking to your doctor about periods

1 Department for Health and Social Care. Women's Health Strategy for England [Internet]. [cited 2024 Jul 1]. Available from: https://www.gov.uk/government/publications/womens-health-strategy-for-england/womens-health-strategy-for-england

2 Department for Health and Social Care. Women's Health Strategy for England [Internet]. [cited 2024 Jul 1]. Available from: https://www.gov.uk/government/publications/womens-health-strategy-for-england/womens-health-strategy-for-england

3 The Food Medic. Perceptions of the menstrual cycle and impact on quality of life, employment, and relationships. [Internet]. 2024 Oct. Available from: https://www.thefoodmedic.co.uk/

4 Johnson A, Thompson R, Nickel B, Shih P, Hammarberg K, Copp T. Websites Selling Direct-to-Consumer Anti-Mullerian Hormone Tests. *JAMA Netw Open*. 2023 Aug 1;6(8):e2330192.

5 Ussher JM, Perz J. Evaluation of the relative efficacy of a couple cognitive-behaviour therapy (CBT) for Premenstrual Disorders (PMDs), in comparison to one-to-one CBT and a wait list control: A randomized controlled trial. *PLoS One*. 2017 Apr 18;12(4):e0175068.

6 Romans SE, Kreindler D, Asllani E, Einstein G, Laredo S, Levitt A, et al. Mood and the Menstrual Cycle. *Psychotherapy and Psychosomatics*. 2012 Nov 6;82(1):53–60.

7 BSI [Internet]. [cited 2024 Jul 1]. BS 30416:2023 Menstruation, Menstrual Health, Menopause. Available from: https://www.bsigroup.com/en-GB/insights-and-media/insights/brochures/bs-30416-menstruation-menstrual-health-and-menopause-in-the-workplace/

8 Levitt RB, Barnack-Tavlaris JL. Addressing Menstruation in the Workplace: The Menstrual Leave Debate. In: Bobel C, Winkler IT, Fahs B, Hasson KA, Kissling EA, Roberts TA, editors. *The Palgrave Handbook of Critical Menstruation Studies*

9 Levitt RB, Barnack-Tavlaris JL. Addressing Menstruation in the Workplace: The Menstrual Leave Debate. In: Bobel C, Winkler IT, Fahs B, Hasson KA, Kissling EA, Roberts TA, editors. *The Palgrave Handbook of Critical Menstruation Studies*

10 The Food Medic. Perceptions of the menstrual cycle and impact on quality of life, employment, and relationships. [Internet]. 2024 Oct. Available from: https://www.thefoodmedic.co.uk/

11 The Food Medic. Perceptions of the menstrual cycle and impact on quality of life, employment, and relationships. [Internet]. 2024 Oct. Available from: https://www.thefoodmedic.co.uk/

12 Okamoto M, Matsumura K, Takahashi A, Kurokawa A, Watanabe Y, Narimatsu H, et al. The Association between Menstrual Symptoms and Presenteeism: A Cross-Sectional Study for Women Working in Central Tokyo. *Int J Environ Res Public Health.* 2024 Mar 8;21(3):313.

Appendix: Common Conditions That Cause Period Problems

1 March WA, Moore VM, Willson KJ, Phillips DIW, Norman RJ, Davies MJ. The prevalence of polycystic ovary syndrome in a community sample assessed under contrasting diagnostic criteria. *Human Reproduction.* 2010 Feb 1;25(2):544–51.

2 Huang A, Brennan K, Azziz R. Prevalence of Hyperandrogenemia in the Polycystic Ovary Syndrome Diagnosed by the NIH 1990 Criteria. *Fertil Steril.* 2010 Apr;93(6):1938–41.

3 Amisi CA. Markers of insulin resistance in Polycystic ovary syndrome women: An update. *World J Diabetes.* 2022 Mar 15;13(3):129–49.

4 Rudnicka E, Suchta K, Grymowicz M, Calik-Ksepka A, Smolarczyk K, Duszewska AM, et al. Chronic Low Grade Inflammation in Pathogenesis of PCOS. *Int J Mol Sci.* 2021 Apr 6;22(7):3789.

5 Wang F, Dou P, Wei W, Liu PJ. Effects of high-protein diets on the cardio-metabolic factors and reproductive hormones of women with polycystic ovary syndrome: a systematic review and meta-analysis. *Nutr Diabetes.* 2024 Feb 29;14(1):1–12.

6 Sørensen LB, Søe M, Halkier KH, Stigsby B, Astrup A. Effects of increased dietary protein-to-carbohydrate ratios in women with polycystic ovary syndrome. *Am J Clin Nutr.* 2012 Jan;95(1):39–48.

7 Kalra B, Kalra S, Sharma JB. The inositols and polycystic ovary syndrome. *Indian J Endocrinol Metab.* 2016;20(5):720–4.

8 Teede HJ, Joham AE, Paul E, Moran LJ, Loxton D, Jolley D, et al. Longitudinal weight gain in women identified with polycystic ovary syndrome:

results of an observational study in young women. *Obesity* (Silver Spring). 2013 Aug;21(8):1526–32.

9 Lim SS, Davies MJ, Norman RJ, Moran LJ. Overweight, obesity and central obesity in women with polycystic ovary syndrome: a systematic review and meta-analysis. *Hum Reprod Update*. 2012;18(6):618–37.

10 Butt MS, Saleem J, Zakar R, Aiman S, Khan MZ, Fischer F. Benefits of physical activity on reproductive health functions among polycystic ovarian syndrome women: a systematic review. *BMC Public Health*. 2023 May 12;23(1):882.

11 Jurczewska J, Ostrowska J, Chełchowska M, Panczyk M, Rudnicka E, Kucharski M, et al. Physical Activity, Rather Than Diet, Is Linked to Lower Insulin Resistance in PCOS Women—A Case-Control Study. *Nutrients*. 2023 Apr 27;15(9):2111.

12 Tsilchorozidou T, Honour JW, Conway GS. Altered Cortisol Metabolism in Polycystic Ovary Syndrome: Insulin Enhances 5α-Reduction But Not the Elevated Adrenal Steroid Production Rates. *The Journal of Clinical Endocrinology & Metabolism*. 2003 Dec 1;88(12):5907–13.

13 Benson S, Arck PC, Tan S, Hahn S, Mann K, Rifaie N, et al. Disturbed stress responses in women with polycystic ovary syndrome. *Psychoneuroendocrinology*. 2009 Jun;34(5):727–35.

14 Moran LJ, March WA, Whitrow MJ, Giles LC, Davies MJ, Moore VM. Sleep disturbances in a community-based sample of women with polycystic ovary syndrome. *Human Reproduction*. 2015 Feb 1;30(2):466–72.

15 Oguz SH, Yildiz BO. An Update on Contraception in Polycystic Ovary Syndrome. *Endocrinol Metab* (Seoul). 2021 Apr;36(2):296–311.

16 de Melo AS, dos Reis RM, Ferriani RA, Vieira CS. Hormonal contraception in women with polycystic ovary syndrome: choices, challenges, and noncontraceptive benefits. *Open Access J Contracept*. 2017 Feb 2;8:13–23.

17 World Health Organization. Endometriosis [Internet]. [cited 2024 Jul 3]. Available from: https://www.who.int/news-room/fact-sheets/detail/endometriosis

18 Cirillo M, Argento FR, Becatti M, Fiorillo C, Coccia ME, Fatini C. Mediterranean Diet and Oxidative Stress: A Relationship with Pain Perception in Endometriosis. *International Journal of Molecular Sciences*. 2023 Jan;24(19):14601.

19 Amini L, Chekini R, Nateghi MR, Haghani H, Jamialahmadi T, Sathyapalan T, et al. The Effect of Combined Vitamin C and Vitamin E

Supplementation on Oxidative Stress Markers in Women with Endometriosis: A Randomized, Triple-Blind Placebo-Controlled Clinical Trial. *Pain Res Manag.* 2021;2021:5529741.

20 Santanam N, Kavtaradze N, Murphy A, Dominguez C, Parthasarathy S. Antioxidant supplementation reduces endometriosis-related pelvic pain in humans. *Transl Res.* 2013 Mar;161(3):189–95.

21 Missmer SA, Chavarro JE, Malspeis S, Bertone-Johnson ER, Hornstein MD, Spiegelman D, et al. A prospective study of dietary fat consumption and endometriosis risk. *Human Reproduction.* 2010 Jun 1;25(6):1528–35.

22 Hopeman MM, Riley JK, Frolova AI, Jiang H, Jungheim ES. Serum Polyunsaturated Fatty Acids and Endometriosis. *Reprod Sci.* 2015 Sep;22(9):1083–7.

23 Mehdizadehkashi A, Rokhgireh S, Tahermanesh K, Eslahi N, Minaeian S, Samimi M. The effect of vitamin D supplementation on clinical symptoms and metabolic profiles in patients with endometriosis. *Gynecol Endocrinol.* 2021 Jul;37(7):640–5.

24 Guo C, Zhang C. Role of the gut microbiota in the pathogenesis of endometriosis: a review. *Front Microbiol.* 2024 Mar 5;15:1363455.

25 Qin R, Tian G, Liu J, Cao L. The gut microbiota and endometriosis: From pathogenesis to diagnosis and treatment. *Front Cell Infect Microbiol.* 2022 Nov 24;12:1069557.

26 Marziali M, Venza M, Lazzaro S, Lazzaro A, Micossi C, Stolfi VM. Gluten-free diet: a new strategy for management of painful endometriosis related symptoms? *Minerva Chir.* 2012 Dec;67(6):499–504.

27 Stephansson O, Falconer H, Ludvigsson JF. Risk of endometriosis in 11 000 women with celiac disease. *Human Reproduction.* 2011 Oct 1;26(10):2896–901.

28 Schink M, Konturek PC, Herbert SL, Renner SP, Burghaus S, Blum S, et al. Different nutrient intake and prevalence of gastrointestinal comorbidities in women with endometriosis. *J Physiol Pharmacol.* 2019 Apr;70(2).

29 Moore JS, Gibson PR, Perry RE, Burgell RE. Endometriosis in patients with irritable bowel syndrome: Specific symptomatic and demographic profile, and response to the low FODMAP diet. *Aust N Z J Obstet Gynaecol.* 2017 Apr;57(2):201–5.

30 Nabi MY, Nauhria S, Reel M, Londono S, Vasireddi A, Elmiry M, et al. Endometriosis and irritable bowel syndrome: A systematic review and meta-analyses. *Front Med* [Internet]. 2022 Jul 25 [cited 2024 Jul 3];9.

Available from: https://www.frontiersin.org/journals/medicine/articles/
10.3389/fmed.2022.914356/full

31 Moore JS, Gibson PR, Perry RE, Burgell RE. Endometriosis in patients
    with irritable bowel syndrome: Specific symptomatic and demographic
    profile, and response to the low FODMAP diet. *Aust N Z J Obstet Gynae-
    col.* 2017 Apr;57(2):201–5.

32 Lacheta J. Uterine adenomyosis: pathogenesis, diagnostics, symptoma-
    tology and treatment. *Ceska Gynekol.* 2019;84(3):240–6.

33 Gunther R, Walker C. Adenomyosis. In: StatPearls [Internet]. Treasure
    Island (FL): StatPearls Publishing; 2024 [cited 2024 Jul 3]. Available from:
    http://www.ncbi.nlm.nih.gov/books/NBK539868/

34 Gunther R, Walker C. Adenomyosis. In: StatPearls [Internet]. Treasure
    Island (FL): StatPearls Publishing; 2024 [cited 2024 Jul 3]. Available from:
    http://www.ncbi.nlm.nih.gov/books/NBK539868/

35 Etrusco A, Barra F, Chiantera V, Ferrero S, Bogliolo S, Evangelisti G, et
    al. Current Medical Therapy for Adenomyosis: From Bench to Bedside.
    Drugs. 2023 Nov 1;83(17):1595–611.

36 nhs.uk [Internet]. 2017 [cited 2024 Jul 3]. Fibroids. Available from: https://
    www.nhs.uk/conditions/fibroids/

37 Eltoukhi HM, Modi MN, Weston M, Armstrong AY, Stewart EA. The
    Health Disparities of Uterine Fibroids for African American Women: A
    Public Health Issue. *Am J Obstet Gynecol.* 2014 Mar;210(3):194–9.

38 Divakar H. Asymptomatic uterine fibroids. *Best Pract Res Clin Obstet
    Gynaecol.* 2008 Aug;22(4):643–54.

39 Wise LA, Radin RG, Palmer JR, Kumanyika SK, Boggs DA, Rosenberg
    L. Intake of fruit, vegetables, and carotenoids in relation to risk of uter-
    ine leiomyoma. *The American Journal of Clinical Nutrition.* 2011 Dec
    1;94(6):1620–31.

40 Wise LA, Radin RG, Palmer JR, Kumanyika SK, Rosenberg L. A Pro-
    spective Study of Dairy Intake and Risk of Uterine Leiomyomata. *Am J
    Epidemiol.* 2010 Jan 15;171(2):221–32.

41 Wise LR, Palmer JL, Harlow B, Spiegelman DA, Stewart EL, Adams-
    Campbell L, et al. Risk of uterine leiomyomata in relation to tobacco,
    alcohol and caffeine consumption in the Black Women's Health Study.
    Hum Reprod. 2004 Aug;19(8):1746–54.

42 Paffoni A, Somigliana E, Vigano' P, Benaglia L, Cardellicchio L,

Pagliardini L, et al. Vitamin D Status in Women With Uterine Leiomyomas. *The Journal of Clinical Endocrinology & Metabo*lism. 2013 Aug 1;98(8):E1374–8.

43 Baird DD, Hill MC, Schectman JM, Hollis BW. Vitamin D and the Risk of Uterine Fibroids. *Epidemiology*. 2013 May;24(3):447.

44 Sabry M, Halder SK, Allah ASA, Roshdy E, Rajaratnam V, Al-Hendy A. Serum vitamin D$_3$ level inversely correlates with uterine fibroid volume in different ethnic groups: a cross-sectional observational study. *IJWH*. 2013 Feb 27;5:93–100.

45 Hodgson R, Bhave Chittawar P, Farquhar C. GnRH agonists for uterine fibroids. *Cochrane Database Syst Rev*. 2017 Oct 29;2017(10):CD012846.

46 Menorrhagia (heavy menstrual bleeding) | Health topics A to Z | CKS | NICE [Internet]. [cited 2024 Jul 2]. Available from: https://cks.nice.org.uk/topics/menorrhagia-heavy-menstrual-bleeding/

47 Kröncke T, David M. Uterine Artery Embolization (UAE) for Fibroid Treatment – Results of the 7th Radiological Gynecological Expert Meeting. RöFo – Fortschritte auf dem Gebiet der Röntgenstrahlen und der bildgebenden Verfahren. 2019 May 28;191:630–4.

48 RCOG. Clinical recommendations on the use of uterine artery embolisation (UAE) in the management of fibroids. 2013.

49 Alkilani YG, Apodaca-Ramos I. Cervical Polyps. In: StatPearls [Internet]. Treasure Island (FL): StatPearls Publishing; 2024 [cited 2024 Jul 3]. Available from: http://www.ncbi.nlm.nih.gov/books/NBK562185/

50 Berceanu C, Cernea N, Căpitănescu RG, Comănescu AC, Paitici Ş, Rotar IC, et al. Endometrial polyps. *Rom J Morphol Embryol*. 2022;63(2):323–34.

51 Practice Committee of the American Society for Reproductive Medicine. Current evaluation of amenorrhea. *Fertil Steril*. 2004 Jul;82(1):266–72.

52 O'Donnell E, Goodman JM, Harvey PJ. Cardiovascular Consequences of Ovarian Disruption: A Focus on Functional Hypothalamic Amenorrhea in Physically Active Women. *The Journal of Clinical Endocrinology & Metabolism*. 2011 Dec 1;96(12):3638–48.

53 Gordon CM, Nelson LM. Amenorrhea and bone health in adolescents and young women. *Curr Opin Obstet Gynecol*. 2003 Oct;15(5):377–84.

54 Marcus MD, Loucks TL, Berga SL. Psychological correlates of functional hypothalamic amenorrhea. *Fertil Steril*. 2001 Aug;76(2):310–6.

55 Shufelt CL, Torbati T, Dutra E. Hypothalamic Amenorrhea and the Long-Term Health Consequences. *Semin Reprod Med*. 2017 May;35(3):256-262.

doi: 10.1055/s-0037-1603581. Epub 2017 Jun 28. PMID: 28658709; PMCID: PMC6374026.

56 Roberts RE, Farahani L, Webber L, Jayasena C. Current understanding of hypothalamic amenorrhoea. *Ther Adv Endocrinol Metab*. 2020 Jul 30;11:2042018820945854.

57 Roberts RE, Farahani L, Webber L, Jayasena C. Current understanding of hypothalamic amenorrhoea. *Ther Adv Endocrinol Metab*. 2020 Jul 30;11:2042018820945854.

Acknowledgements

First and foremost, thank you to *you* – the reader. By picking up this book, you've not only embarked on a journey I know will be helpful but also cast a meaningful vote towards making conversations about the menstrual cycle more mainstream. Your support means more than you know.

To my best friend and fiancé, David – thank you for being my biggest supporter throughout this process. From endless cups of coffee to late-night proofreads and much-needed reassurance, your encouragement has been unwavering. I think it's safe to say you know the content of this book almost as well as I do!

To my manager, Nora Millar – thank you for always championing my work and being at the end of the phone when I need you. And to Carly Cook, my wonderful book agent – since our first book together in 2016, every step of the way with you has been a joy. Your guidance and friendship have made this journey both a success and a lot of fun!

Jodie Lancet-Grant and the Bluebird team – Amy, Annie, and everyone else – thank you for taking a chance on me and making me feel so welcome within the Bluebird family. I'm so proud of the work we have done together.

To my family and friends – thank you for your patience while I buried myself away for months. Your words of encouragement kept me going.

To the brilliant experts who contributed to this work – Dr Thivi Maruthappu, Michelle Carroll, Maeve Hanan and Elle Kelly – your insights have made this book even richer. And to my wonderful research assistant, Bríd Ní Dhonnabháin – thank you for your dedication and for helping me pull everything together. This book would not have been possible without you!

Finally, to my clients and amazing social media community – this book exists because of you! Your engagement, enthusiasm and voices have made this opportunity possible, and I'm endlessly grateful.